Biomedical Imaging

Edited by

Youxin Mao

Biomedical Imaging
Edited by Youxin Mao

Republished by InTech
Janeza Trdine 9, 51000 Rijeka, Croatia

Technical Editor Melita Horvat

Cover Designer Dino Smrekar

Additional hard copies can be obtained from orders@intechopen.com

Biomedical Imaging,
Edited by Youxin Mao
p. cm.
ISBN 978-953-307-071-1

For EU product safety concerns:
IN TECH d.o.o., Prolaz Marije Krucifikse Kozulić 3, 51000 Rijeka, Croatia,
info@intechopen.com or visit our website at intechopen.com.

Meet the editor

Youxin Mao received her BS degree in physics and her MS degree in electronics science from Nankai University, China, in 1982 and 1985, respectively. She received her PhD in optoelectronics from Lancaster University, United Kingdom, in 1995. She was later a research associate with Lancaster University and an NSERC visiting fellowship with the National Research Council in Canada. As a research scientist, she worked in an exploratory research and development group with JDS Uniphase from 1999 to 2003. She has been working on optical coherence tomography in Nankai University and the University of Toronto since 2003. She is currently a research officer for the National Research Council of Canada. Her research interests include optical coherence tomography, high speed and high power wavelength swept laser, and ultra small optical fiber probes.

Preface

Biomedical imaging is becoming an indispensable branch within bioengineering. This research field has recent expanded due to the requirement of high-level medical diagnostics and rapid development of interdisciplinary modern technologies. This book is designed to present the most recent advances in instrumentation, methods, and image processing as well as clinical applications in important areas of biomedical imaging. This book provides broad coverage of the field of biomedical imaging, with particular attention to an engineering viewpoint.

Chapter one introduces a 3D volumetric image registration technique. The foundations of the volumetric image visualization, classification and registration are discussed in detail. Although this highly accurate registration technique is established from three phantom experiments (CT, MRI and PET/CT), it applies to all imaging modalities. Optical imaging has recently experienced explosive growth due to the high resolution, noninvasive or minimally invasive nature and cost-effectiveness of optical coherence modalities in medical diagnostics and therapy. Chapter two demonstrates a fiber catheter-based complex swept-source optical coherence tomography system. Swept-source, quadrature interferometer, and fiber probes used in optical coherence tomography system are described in details. The results indicate that optical coherence tomography is a potential imaging tool for *in vivo* and real-time diagnosis, visualization and treatment monitoring in clinic environments. Brain computer interfaces have attracted great interest in the last decade. Chapter three introduces brain imaging and machine learning for brain computer interface. Non-invasive approaches for brain computer interface are the main focus. Several techniques have been proposed to measure relevant features from EEG or MRI signals and to decode the brain targets from those features. Such techniques are reviewed in the chapter with a focus on a specific approach. The basic idea is to make the comparison between a BCI system and the use of brain imaging in medical applications. Texture analysis methods are useful for discriminating and studying both distinct and subtle textures in multi-modality medical images. In chapter four, texture analysis is presented as a useful computational method for discriminating between pathologically different regions on medical images. This is particularly important given that biomedical image data with near isotropic resolution is becoming more common in clinical environments.

The goal of this book is to provide a wide-ranging forum in the biomedical imaging field that integrates interdisciplinary research and development of interest to scientists, engineers, teachers, students, and clinical providers. This book is suitable as both a professional reference and as a text for a one-semester course for biomedical engineers or medical technology students.

Youxin Mao
Institute for Microstructural Science,
National Research Council Canada

Contents

1

Volumetric Image Registration of Multi-modality Images of CT, MRI and PET

Guang Li and Robert W. Miller
National Cancer Institute, National Institutes of Health
Bethesda, Maryland,USA

1. Introduction

1.1 Biomedical Imaging of Multimodality

Three-dimensional (3D) biomedical imaging starts from computed tomography (CT) in 1960's-1970's (Cormack, 1963, Hounsfield, 1973) followed by magnetic resonance imaging (MRI) in 1970's (Lauterbur, 1973, Garroway et al, 1974, Mansfield & Maudsley, 1977). These anatomical imaging techniques are based on physical features of a patient's anatomy, such as linear attenuation coefficient or electromagnetic interaction and relaxation. 3D biological imaging (molecular imaging or functional imaging), such as positron emission tomography (PET) and single photon emission computed tomography (SPECT), was also developed in mid 1970's (Ter-Pogossian, et al, 1975, Phelps, et al, 1975). They detect biological features using a molecular probe, labelled with either a positron emitter or a gamma emitter, to target a molecular, cellular or physiological event, process or product. So, the x-ray/γ-ray intensity from a particular anatomical site is directly related to the concentration of the radio-labelled molecular marker. Therefore, a biological event will be imaged in 3D space. Since the concept of hybrid PET/CT scanner was introduced (Beyer, et al, 2000), the co-registration of biological image with anatomical image offers both biological and anatomical information in space, assuming that there is no patient's motion between and during the two image acquisitions. Other combined scanners, such as SPECT/CT and PET/MRI, have also been developed (Cho, et al, 2007, Bybel, et al, 2008, Chowdhury & Scarsbrook, 2008). Registration of biological and anatomical images at acquisition or post acquisition provides multi-dimensional information on patient's disease stage (Ling, et al, 2000), facilitating lesion identification for diagnosis and target delineation for treatment.

In radiological clinic, although a particular imaging modality may be preferable to diagnose a particular disease, multimodality imaging has been increasingly employed for early diagnosing malignant lesion (Osman, et al, 2003), coronary artery diseases (Elhendy, et al 2002), and other diseases. Use of biological imaging enhances the success rate of correct diagnosis, which is necessary for early, effective treatment and ultimate cure.

In radiation therapy clinic, multi-modality imaging is increasingly employed to assist target delineation and localization, aiming to have a better local control of cancer (Nestle, et al,

2009). Radiation therapy (RT) contains three basic components: treatment simulation, treatment planning and treatment delivery (Song & Li, 2008). Simulation is to imaging a patient at treatment condition for planning, based on which the treatment is delivered. In image-based planning, multimodality images, including CT, MRI and PET, can be registered and used to define the target volume and location within the anatomy (Schad et al, 1987, Chen & Pelizzari, 1989). In image-guided delivery, on-site imaging which provides patient's positioning image, is used to register to the planning CT image for accurate patient setup, so that the target is treated as planned (Jaffray, et al, 2007).

Therefore, in both diagnostic and therapeutic imaging, image registration is critical for a successful clinical application. Beyond the 3D space, 4D (3D+time) biomedical imaging has become an emerging clinical research field, and some procedures have been adopted in the clinic, such as 4DCT (Li et al, 2008a). Motion is inevitably present during imaging as well as therapeutic processes, including respiratory, cardiac, digestive and muscular motions, causing image blurring and target relocation. 4D medical imaging aims to minimize the motion artefact and 4DRT aims to track and compensate for the target motion. Facing the challenge of patient's motion and change along the time, deformable image registration has been intensively studied (Hill, et al, 2001, Pluim et al, 2003, Li et al, 2008b). Although it remains as challenging topic, it will be only discussed briefly where it is needed, as it is not the main focus of this chapter.

1.2 Manual Image Registration

Manual or interactive image registration is guided by visual indication of image alignment. The conventional visual representation of an 3D images is 2D-based, three orthogonal planar views of cross-section of the volumetric image (West, et al, 1997, Fitzpatrick, et al, 1998). Here the discussion will be focused on anatomy-based image registration, rather than fiducial-based (such as superficial or implanted markers) or coordinate-based (such as combined PET/CT system). All clinical treatment planning systems utilize this visual representation for checking and adjusting the alignment of two images. In details, there are several means to achieve the visual alignment verification: (1) the chess-box display of two images in alternate boxes; (2) the simultaneous display of two mono-coloured images; and (3) the superimposed display of the two images with an adjustable weighting factor. Fig. 1 illustrates the first two of the three basic visualization methods.

The 2D visual-based fusion technique has been developed, validated and adopted for biomedical research as well as clinical practice (Hibbard, et al, 1987, Chen, et al, 1987, Hibbard & Hawkins, 1988, Pelizzari, et al, 1989, Toga & Banerjee, 1993, Maintz & Viergever, 1998, Hill, et al, 2001). Throughout the past three decades, this technique has evolved and become a well developed tool to align 3D images in the clinic. Multi-modality image registration is required (Schad et al, 1987, Pelizzari, et al, 1989) as more medical imaging is available to the clinic. However, reports have shown that this well established technique may suffer from (1) large intra- and inter-observer variability; (2) the dependency of user's cognitive ability; (3) limited precision by the resolution of imaging and image display; and (4) time consuming in verifying and adjusting alignment in three series of planar views in three orthogonal directions (Fitzpatrick, et al, 1998, Vaarkamp, 2001). These findings have become a concern whether this 2D visual-based fusion technique with an accuracy of 1-3 mm and time requirement of 15-20 minutes is sufficiently accurate and fast to meet the clinical challenges of increasing utilization of multi-modality images in planning, increasing adoption of image-guided delivery, and increasing throughput of patient treatments.

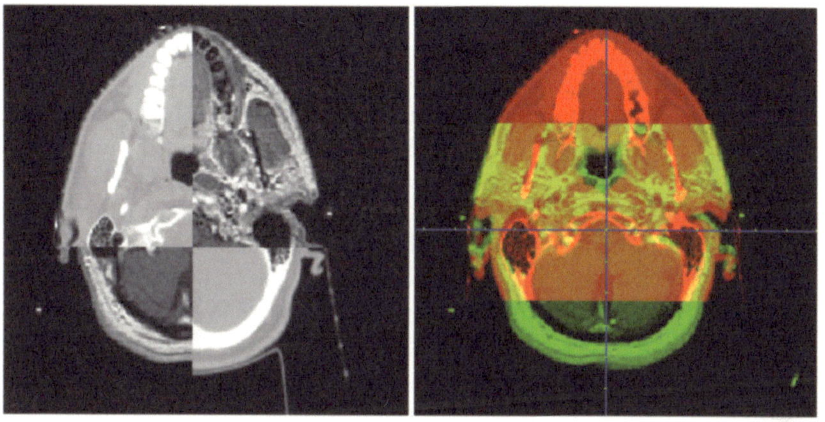

Fig. 1. Illustration of two common means of image alignment based on 2D planar views (Only one of the axial slices is shown, and the sagittal and coronal series are not shown).

The 3D visual representation or volumetric visualization (Udupa, 1999, Schroeder, et al, 2004) has recently been applied to evaluate the volumetric alignment of two or more 3D images (Xie, et al, 2004, Li, et al, 2005, 2007, 2008b and 2008c). This 3D volumetric image registration (3DVIR) technique aims to solve most of the problems associated with the conventional 2D fusion technique by providing a fundamentally different, volumetric visual representation of multimodality images. This volumetric technique has been successfully designed, developed and validated, while it is still relatively new to the medical field and has not been widely adopted as an alternative (superior) to the conventional 2D visual fusion technique. Two of the major obstacles for the limited clinical applications are that (1) from 2D to 3D visualization, the clinical practitioners have to be retrained to adapt themselves to this new technique, and (2) this technique has not yet been commercially available to the clinic.

1.3 Automatic Image Registration

Automatic image registration can improve the efficiency and accuracy of the visual-based manual fusion technique. There are three major components in any automatic image registration, including (1) registration criterion; (2) transformation and interpolation; and (3) optimization. These three components are independent of one another, so that they can be freely recombined for an optimal outcome in a particular clinical application. Here again, the discussion will focus on anatomy-based rigid image registration, rather than fiducial-based or coordinate-based registration.

Before mutual information criterion (negative cost function) was developed in 1995 (Viola & Wells, 1995), other algorithms were utilized, such as Chamfer surface matching criterion (Borgefors, 1988, van Herk & Kooy, 1994) or voxel intensity similarity criterion (Venot, et al, 1984). Mutual information is fundamentally derived from information theory and has been extensively discussed in the literature (Hill, et al, 2001, Pluim, et al, 2003). It is worthwhile to mention that among existing criteria the common features in two different modality images are best described by the mutual information, which can serve as the registration cost function for maximization to achieve multi-modality image registration.

The transformation and interpolation are mathematical operations of the images. For rigid image registration, only six degrees of freedom (three rotational and three translational) are in the transformation and the transformed voxels are assigned through interpolation (linear, nearest neighbour, or Spline). For deformable image registration, however, the number of degree of freedom is dramatically increased, since all voxels are allowed to move (deform) independently and therefore the number of variables would be up to three times of the total number of voxels in an image. As a consequence, the performance of deformable image registration becomes one of the bottlenecks, despite that several simplified algorithms have been studied to address this challenging problem (Pluim et al, 2003, Li et al, 2008a & 2008b).

The optimization process is to minimize (or maximize) the cost function (or to refine the registration criterion) until a pre-determined threshold is met. There are many established algorithms available, including Gradient descent, Simplex, Genetics, and Simulated Annealing (Kirkpatrick et al, 1983, Goldberg et al, 1989, Snyman, 2005). The performance of these algorithms is evaluated based on their ability and speed to find a global minimum (or maximum), avoiding local traps, which will lead to a faulty result. Therefore, any automatic image registration must be verified visually to ensure a correct or acceptable result.

Image registration based on anatomic features has a fundamental assumption, which is the identical underlying anatomy in different imaging modalities. In other words, motion and deformation of the anatomy between scans will post uncertainty to rigid image registration. For rigid anatomy, such as head, the accuracy of the automatic registration based on maximization of mutual information (MMI) can reach sub-mm scale. Clinical images of a patient often contain anatomical variations, resulting in sub-optimal registration results, which must be visually verified and adjusted to a clinically accepted level. Manual adjustment is mostly based on the 2D fusion technique, together with anatomical and physiological knowledge. Therefore this process inherits the drawbacks of the 2D fusion technique and degrades the accuracy of automatic registration.

1.4 Hybrid Image Registration with Segmentation and Visualization

Anatomy-based image registration can be further categorized as (1) using all voxels within the field of view (the anatomy and surrounding objects), such as MMI and greyscale similarity, and (2) using selected anatomical landmarks, such as Chamfer surface (van Herk & Kooy 1994) and manual registration (Fitzpatrick, et al, 1998, Vaarkamp, 2001, Li, et al, 2005 & 2008c). In most medical images, some anatomies are more reliable to serve as landmarks than others, because of anatomical rigidity, less motion artefacts, and/or sufficient image contrast. Therefore, evenly utilizing the entire anatomy, including medical devices present in the images, is good for automation, but may not be optimal for achieving the most accurate and reliable result. In contrast, a feature-based image registration with full or semi automation is sometimes preferable, especially for clinical cases with high degree of

difficulty or with high accuracy requirement. We have found that pairing automatic MMI registration and the 3DVIR serves the best in terms of registration speed and outcome.
The advantage of hybridized image registration is that it will take the advantage of multiple image processing techniques. Image segmentation/classification can extract more reliable features from the original image to enhance image registration with the more informative features. Image (volumetric) visualization can enhance image registration, if a classified reliable anatomy is visualized and utilized as the registration landmark. Therefore, hybrid image registration remains a focus of clinical research (Li, et al, 2008b). Although feature extraction is often application specific and few algorithms can be employed across the spectrum of all imaging modalities, hybrid image registration, such as the 3DVIR, has shown its promise to resolve particular clinical problems that require high accuracy.

1.5 Visual Verification of Registration

Although automatic rigid image registration using mutual information has been widely accepted in radiotherapy clinic, the necessity of visual verification of the result prior to clinical use will never change. Several causes for a sub-optimal automatic registration result include (1) changes in patient's anatomy between scans; (2) incomplete or insufficient anatomy, especially in biological images; (3) poor image quality, and (4) incorrect (local traps) or insensitive (flat surface) registration outcomes. Visual verification and adjustment allow user to check and correct any misalignment in the auto-registered images.

As discussed above, the only viable, visual method in the current clinic is the 2D-based fusion technique, which possesses many drawbacks, including observer dependency, error prone and time consuming (Vaarkamp, 2001, Li, et al, 2005). Therefore, no matter how accurate an automatic registration result would be, once it is adjusted with the manual fusion tool, the uncertainty of the result will fall back to that of the manual registration (±1-3 mm). Thereby, the mismatch of accuracy between the automatic and manual registration will diminish the accuracy advantage of the automatic registration. In other words, the gain in reliability via visual verification and adjustment may sacrifice the accuracy.

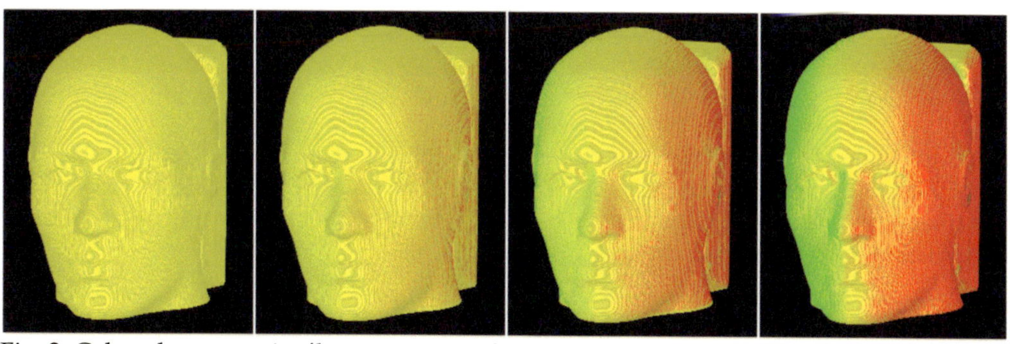

Fig. 2. Colour homogeneity/heterogeneity of two overlaid, identical images (red and green) with misalignment of 0.0, 0.2, 0.5 and 1.0 voxel (mm) from left to right using the 3DVIR. The "elevation contour pattern" is due to limited imaging resolution and should be ignored.

Recently, reports have shown that the 3DVIR technique is superior to the conventional 2D visual fusion method, in terms of improved registration performance as well as high accuracy (±0.1 mm) that matches or exceeds that of automatic registration (Li, et al, 2008c). Therefore, combining an automatic registration with the 3DVIR technique seems a desirable alternative to overcome the limitations of the 2D fusion method, providing a solution for registration verification with preserved or even enhanced accuracy, as shown in Fig. 2.

2. 3D Volumetric Image Registration (3DVIR)

2.1 Volumetric Image Visualization and Classification

Volumetric image visualization is an advanced image rendering technique, which generally offers two different approaches: (1) object-order volume rendering and (2) image-order volume rendering (Schroeder et al, 2004). Based on the camera (view point of an observer) settings, the former renders in the order of voxels stored while the latter is based on ray casting, which is employed in the 3DVIR technique.

Ray casting determines the value of each pixel in the image plane by passing a ray from the current camera view through the pixel into the scene, or the image volume in this case. An array of parallel rays is used to cover the entire image plane, as shown in Fig. 3. Along each ray, all encountered voxels will contribute to the appearance of the pixel through colour blending until the accumulated transparency (alpha, or A) becomes unity. Here an advanced voxel format is employed with four components (RGBA), representing red, green, blue, and alpha. The colour blending of the pixel can follow any mathematical formula. In the 3DVIR technique, however, the following equations are used to mimic the physical appearance of an image volume with controllable transparency:

$$
\begin{aligned}
R^{i+1}_{Accum} &= R^{i}_{Accum} + (1.0 - A^{i}_{Accum}) \cdot R^{i} \cdot A^{i} \\
G^{i+1}_{Accum} &= G^{i}_{Accum} + (1.0 - A^{i}_{Accum}) \cdot G^{i} \cdot A^{i} \\
B^{i+1}_{Accum} &= B^{i}_{Accum} + (1.0 - A^{i}_{Accum}) \cdot B^{i} \cdot A^{i}
\end{aligned}
\tag{1}
$$

$$
A^{i+1}_{Accum} = A^{i}_{Accum} + (1.0 - A^{i}_{Accum}) \cdot A^{i} \tag{2}
$$

where the superscripts i and i+1 represent the two consecutive steps along the ray path and the subscript represents accumulative values, which are the blended RGBA values for the pixels up to the steps i or i+1. For any voxel with $A^i = 0$ (totally transparent), it does not contribute to the pixel. For any voxel with $A^i = 1$ (totally opaque) or $A^i_{Accum} = 1$ (becoming opaque after step i), all voxels afterward along the ray are invisible as they no longer contribute to the blended pixel in the image plane.

Four lookup tables (LUTs) over the image histogram are utilized to control the voxel RGBA value based on voxel greyscale. The transparency A-LUT in the histogram can be used for image classification, which relies on large greyscale gradient at interface of an anatomy, as shown in Fig. 4. Mono-coloured image can also be created using the RGB LUT(s), such as a primary colour (e.g., red: R; G=B=0), a secondary colour (e.g., yellow: R=G; B=0), or a tertiary colour (e.g., white: R=G=B). These pseudo-colour representations of the volumetric images enable visual-based image alignment using volumetric anatomical landmarks. In practice, we recommend to use the three primary colours (RGB), so that the origin of a voxel is instantly identifiable without interference from synthesized secondary colours. The white colour should be used for the 4th image, which can be identified by its colour appearance and by toggling on and off this image, since white can also result from overlay of the other three images (RGB). Up to four volumetric images can be rendered simultaneously via the ray casting and they can be individually turned on or off as desired.

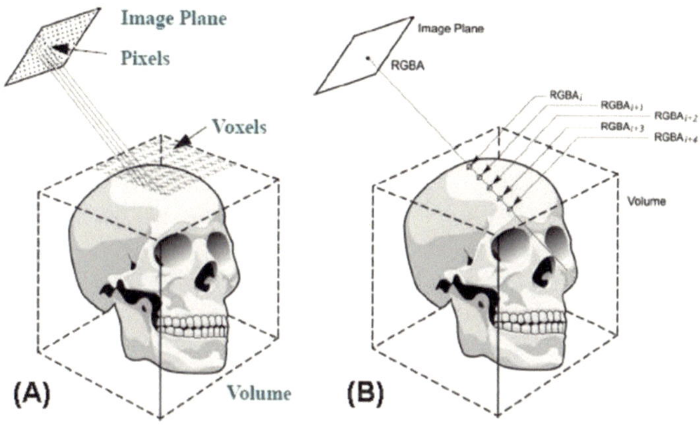

Fig. 3. Illustration of ray casting and RGBA blending for volumetric image rendering. (taken from Li, et al, JACMP, 2008c)

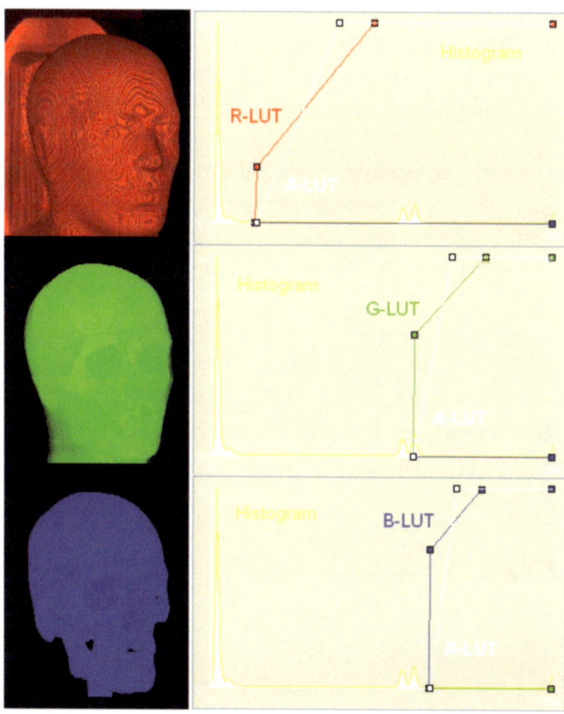

Fig. 4. Illustration of image classification using the transparency lookup table, which is the sophisticated form of window-level function. The skin (red) and bone (blue) are shown.

2.2 Visual Criterion of the Volumetric Image Registration

When two mono-coloured, identical images are overlaid in space, the colour blending of the equal-intensity (greyscale) voxels produce a homogeneously coloured image based on the colour synthesis rule of light. For instance, the overlay of equally-weighted red and green will result in a yellow appearance. Therefore, an ideal image alignment will show a perfect homogeneous colour distribution on a volumetric anatomic landmark. On the other hand, any misalignment of two rigid images will show various degrees of colour heterogeneity distributed on the volumetric landmark, as shown in Fig. 2. Therefore, the homogeneity of colour distribution on volumetric anatomical landmarks has been established as the visual registration criterion (Li et al, 2005).

It is worthwhile to mention that the greyscale of the mono-coloured image is controlled by the RGB-LUT(s), which have a value of 0 to 1 (dark to bright). Such mono-colour greyscale is important to show the stereo-spatial effect; without it (e.g., a flat LUT=constant) the landmarks are hard to be identified as 3D objects, except for the peripheral region in the 2D image plane. So, an uneven greyscale should be used in the RGB-LUT(s), as shown in Fig. 4, and the colour greyscale variation should not be regarded as colour heterogeneity.

2.3 Quantitative Criterion of the Volumetric Registration

Quantitatively, the above visual-based criterion for volumetric alignment can be directly translated into a mathematical expression. By definition, the homogeneity of the colour distribution on a given volumetric anatomical landmark should have minimal variance in the visible voxel intensity difference (VVID) between any two mono-coloured imaging modalities, namely a random colour distribution (or "snow pattern"). In other words, a misalignment should appear to have a systematic, colour-biased distribution (or global alignment aberration), which should show a large variation of the VVID.

With uniform sampling across the image plane, about 4% of the pixels are sufficient for evaluating the registration criterion. The visible voxels on the anatomical landmark can be traced along the ray automatically using a special algorithm under the ray casting rendering scheme (Li, et al, 2008c). Mathematically, for any visible voxel (i), the VVID is defined:

$$\Delta I_i = I_i^A - I_i^B \tag{3}$$

where I_i^A and I_i^B (<256 = 8 bits) are the VVI from images A and B, respectively. For all sampled voxels, the variance of the VVID is:

$$VAR = \sum_{i=1}^{N} \frac{(\Delta I_i - \Delta I)^2}{N} = \sum_{i=1}^{N} \frac{(I_i^A - I_i^B - \Delta I)^2}{N} \tag{4}$$

where $\Delta I = \sum (\Delta I_i / N)$ represents the average of the VVID and N is the total number of the voxels sampled, excluding completely transparent rays. In case of two identical images, the variance of VVID approaches zero at the perfect alignment, as shown in Fig. 2.

In multi-modality image registration, the average voxel intensity of an anatomical landmark can differ substantially between modalities, so a baseline correction is required. Therefore, a modality baseline weighting factor (R) is introduced as:

$$R = \frac{\overline{I^A}}{\overline{I^B}} = \sum_{i=1}^{N} I_i^A \Big/ \sum_{i=1}^{N} I_i^B \tag{5}$$

and the modified variance ($mVAR$) with baseline correction is defined as:

$$mVAR = \sum_{i=1}^{N} \frac{(\Delta I_i * - \Delta I *)^2}{N} = \sum_{i=1}^{N} \frac{((I_i^A / R) - I_i^B - \Delta I *)^2}{N} \tag{6}$$

where $\Delta I^* = \sum (\Delta I_i * / N)$ is the average of modified VVID $(\Delta I_i * = I_i^A / R - I_i^B)$. This quantitative measure, when minimized, indicates an optimal image alignment from a single viewing point.

To evaluate the volumetric image alignment, multiple views (e.g., six views) should be used to provide a comprehensive evaluation, although single view is sufficient for fine tuning around the optimal alignment (Li, et al, 2007). A simple or weighted average of the mVAR from different views can serve as the cost function with a high confidence level, as each individual $mVAR$ can be cross-verified with each other. In addition, the quantitative criteria can be verified by visual examination with similar sensitivity, avoiding local minima.

2.4 Advantages of Volumetric Image Registration

With both the visual and the quantitative registration criteria, this interactive registration technique can be readily upgraded into an automatic registration technique, which is an on-going investigation. Currently, the quantitative criterion can be applied in the fine-tuning stage of image registration, minimizing the potential user dependency. As a comparison, the 2D visual based fusion technique does not have such quantitative evaluation on the alignment. The precision for the rigid transformation and linear interpolation is set at 0.1 voxel (~mm), although it is not limited, matching the high spatial sensitivity of the 3DVIR technique, as shown in Fig. 2. Similar accuracy has been found between the visual and quantitative criteria (will be discussed in the next section), allowing visual verification of the potential automatic 3DVIR with the consistent accuracy and reliability.

The design of the volumetric image registration enables user to simultaneously process up to four images, meeting the challenges of increasing imaging modalities used in the clinic and eliminating potential error propagation from separated registrations. The flowchart of the volumetric image registration process is demonstrated in Fig. 5. The image buffer (32 bits) is divided into 4 fields for 4 images (8 bits or 256 greyscale each). Transformation operation can be applied to any of the four image fields for alignment and all four images are rendered together for real-time visual display, supported by a graph processing unit

(GPU), or volume rendering video card (volumePro, Terarecon, Inc.). The alignment evaluation is based on multiple views by rotating the image volumes with mouse control in real-time. If the criterion is not satisfied, more transformations will be done iteratively until the alignment is achieved.

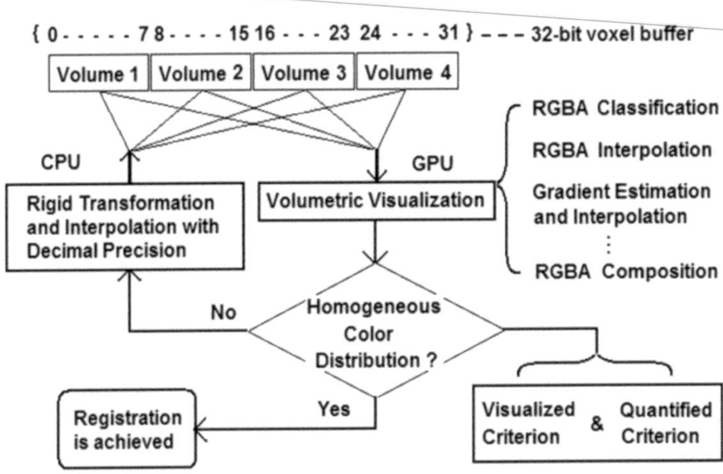

Fig. 5. Illustration of the working flow of the volume-view-guided image registration. (taken from Li, et al, JACMP, 2008c)

3. Accuracy of 3D Volumetric Image Registration

3.1 Sensitivity of Volumetric Registration Criteria

The colour homogeneity (or variance of the VVID) is defined in a new dimension beyond the 3D volumetric space, in which the image alignment is examined. The sensitivity of the 3DVIR criteria is enhanced by visual amplification of the alignment on classified volumetric landmarks, where a large greyscale gradient exists at the interface. For instances, the interfaces of skin/air and bone/soft tissue possess very large intensity gradient. In CT images, the greyscale at these interfaces spans half of the entire intensity range (-1000 HU to +1000 HU). Mathematically, this can be expressed as:

$$dVVI >> dD \quad or \quad \frac{dVVI}{dD} >> 1 \tag{7}$$

where dVVI is the intensity differential resulting from dD, which is the spatial displacement within a voxel (~1 mm). So, the VVID (the difference of the VVIs in two images) should possess a large change upon a small spatial shift. In other words, a small spatial difference will be amplified as a large VVID or colour inhomogeneity. This signal amplification nature is the foundation for the 3DVIR to become extremely sensitive.

The visual detection limit has been evaluated using eight clinical professionals, who were asked to identify colour inhomogeneity or homogeneity for given sets of volumetric images with or without spatial misalignments. Twelve images with known shifts of 0.0, 0.1 and 0.2 unit (mm or degree) were shown to the observers, and the success rates are 94%, 80% and 100%, respectively, as shown in Figs. 2 and 6. The visual detection limit is determined to be 0.1° or 0.1 mm, where the colour homogeneity/inhomogeneity on the skin landmark starts to become indistinguishable to some of the observers. Half of these observers saw such volumetric images for the first time and visual training could improve the success rate.

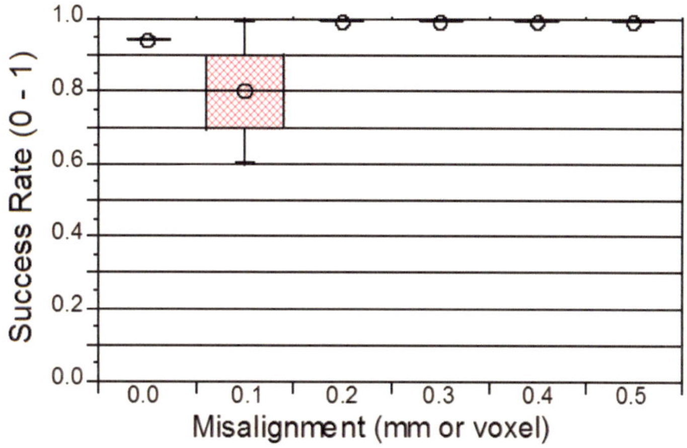

Fig. 6. Success rate of identification of colour inhomogeneity or homegeneity in misaligned or aligned images. The visual detection limits of 0.1° and 0.1 mm are determined.

Quantitatively, the detection limit was evaluated using plots of the VVID vs. misalignment from different viewing angles. U-shaped curves are observed with the nadir at the perfect alignment, as shown in Fig. 7. The result is generally consistent with the visual detection limit of 0.1° and 0.1 mm, with higher precision. For single modality, the variance in Eq. 4 is used and for dual modality, the modified variance in Eq. 6 is used. Although the U-curves become shallow when different imaging modalities are processed, correct image registration (from single or hybrid image scanner) is achieved.

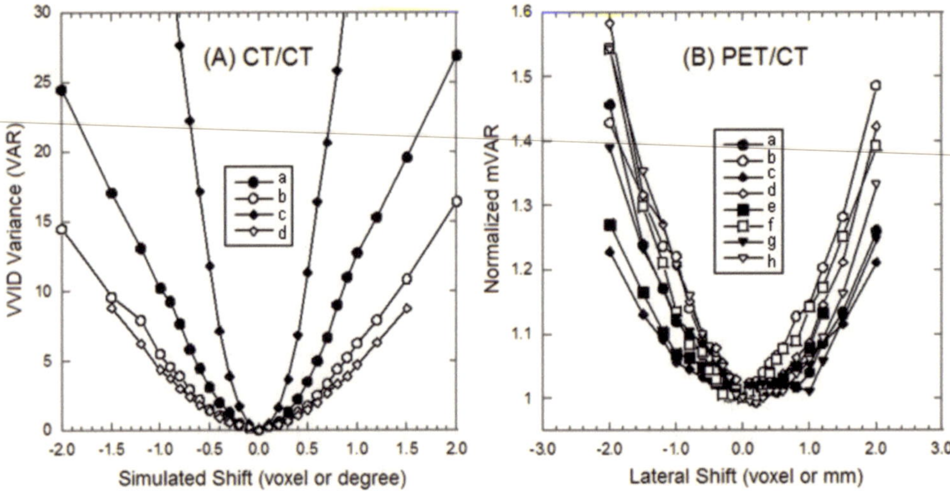

Fig. 7. Alignment of phantom images with translational or rotational shifts in two views (frontal: solid and sagittal: open) using the quantitative criterion and surface landmark. (taken from Li, et al, JACMP, 2008c)

3.2 Accuracy of Volumetric Image Registration

Three phantom experiments have been performed to determine the registration accuracy (Li, et al, 2008c). The phantoms are shown in Fig. 8. Three physical shifts with interval of 5.0±0.1 mm are applied to the phantom between scans, and the acquired images are aligned using the 3DVIR with image shifts to correct the physical misalignments. The physical shifts and image shifts are compared, showing a discrepancy (the accuracy) within 0.1 mm.

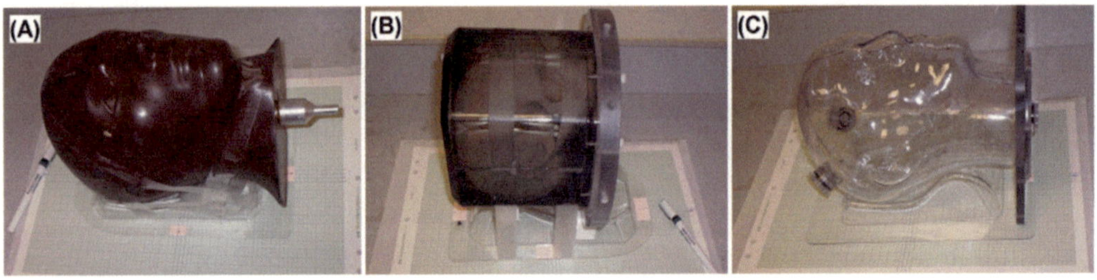

Fig. 8. Three anthromorphic head phantoms for CT (A), MRI (B), and PET/CT (C) imaging.

The experimental results, as shown in Table 1, indicate a discrepancy of 0.02±0.09 mm between and registration results lateral shifts for CT images. The 3DVIR is highly sensitive to small misalignment: it can detect the longitudinal couch positioning uncertainty (0.3±0.2 mm), which is within the manufacturer's technical specification (<0.5 mm). For MRI images, the registration landmark of the brain is used, which is defined as the innar surface of the skull. Similar accuracy (0.03±0.07 mm) is obtained.

Physical Shifts (mm)	Registration Shifts (mm)				Statistical Analysis (mm)		
X_{Exp}	X_1	X_2	X_3	X_4	X_{Avg}	X_{Exp} - X_{Avg}	St.dev.
5.0±0.1	4.92	4.92	4.99	5.07	4.98	0.02	0.08
10.0±0.1	9.92	10.14	9.99	9.99	10.01	-0.01	0.09
15.0±0.1	14.91	14.91	14.91	15.08	14.95	0.05	0.10
Average						**0.02**	**0.09**

Table 1. Accuracy of the volumetric registration by comparison with physical shift (lateral).

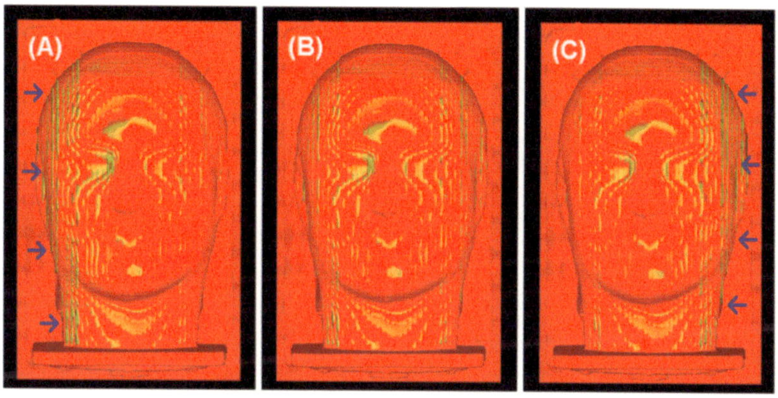

Fig. 9. Volumetric image registration of PET/CT phantom images with -0.5, 0.0 and 0.5 mm misalignments. The arrows show the colour inhomogeneity in the images. (taken from Li, et al, JACMP, 2008c)

For PET/CT images, the "skin" landmark is employed and the PET skin is determined in reference to the CT skin with similar image volume (both are shown for alignment). The visual and the quantitative criteria produce a similar accuracy, 0.03±0.35 mm and 0.05±0.09 mm, respectively, but the latter has higher precision. Supprisingly, this 0.1 mm accuracy is the same as that of anatomical image registration. This modality independency is because the alignment is assessed in the 4th dimension beyond 3D space, independent of (or insensitive to) image resolution and display resolution. Fig. 9 shows the PET/CT image alignment of the phantom with or without lateral misalignment.

3.3 Comparison with Other Registration Techniques

Two clinical viable image registration techniques are compared with the 3DVIR technique based on cranial images of 14 patients, including (1) the 2D visual-based fusion with three orthogonal planar views and (2) the automatic image registration with maximization of mutual information. These two registrations are separately performed based on their own criteria, and then the registered images are evaluated using the 3DVIR criteria for verification and adjustment, if a misalignment is identified (Li, et al, 2005).

The 2D visual-based fusion technique has been reported to have large inter-/intra-observer variations, single pixel precision, and time-consuming (Fitzpatrick, et al, 1998, Vaarkamp, 2001). Our study indicates that the 2D technique tends to produce a sizable, unrealized registration error of 1.8°±1.2° and 2.0±1.3 mm, as shown in Table 2. For automatic MMI registration, the results are consistent with the 3DVIR within a tolerance of 0.5°±0.7° and 0.3±0.5 mm. But, the automatic registration fails in two occasions, as shown in Table 3. On the skin landmark, the 3DVIR criteria indicate a small misalignment in some of the MMI results, shown in Table 3.

Patients (Images) *	Rotational Correction (°)		Translational Correction (mm)	
	$\Sigma\|\delta\|/3$	$(\Sigma\delta^2)^{1/2}$	$\Sigma\|\delta\|/3$	$(\Sigma\delta^2)^{1/2}$
1 (CT/MR_T1-Flair)	0	0.00	1	1.73
2 (CT/MR_T2)	0.67	1.41	1.33	2.45
3 (CT/MR_T1-Flair)	1	3.00	1	3.00
4 (CT/MR_T1-Gd)	0.33	1.00	0.33	1.00
5 (CT/MR_T1-Gd)	0.67	2.00	0.33	1.00
6 (CT/MR_T1-3D)	1	2.24	0.67	2.00
7 (CT/MR_T1-Flair)	0.67	2.00	0.33	1.00
8 (CT/MR_T1-Gd)	0.33	1.00	0.33	1.00
9 (CT/MR_T2)	1	2.24	1.67	4.12
10(CT/MR_T1-Flair)	1	1.73	0.33	1.00
11(CT/MR_T1-3D)	1	2.24	1.33	4.00
12(CT/MR_T1-Flair)	0	0.00	0	0.00
13(CT/MR_T1-Gd)	2	4.47	1.67	3.32
14(CT/MR_T1-Gd)	0.67	1.41	1.33	2.45
Ave ($\Sigma\|\delta\|/N$)	0.7	1.8	0.8	2.0
Std Dev (σ)	0.5	1.2	0.6	1.3

Table 2. Misalignment of the 2D fusion of patient's CT/MR images, corrected by the 3DVIR (taken from Li, et al, IJROBP, 2005, with permission)

Patients (Images) *	Rotational Correction (°)		Translational Correction (mm)	
	$\Sigma\|\delta\|/3$	$(\Sigma\delta^2)^{1/2}$	$\Sigma\|\delta\|/3$	$(\Sigma\delta^2)^{1/2}$
1 (CT/MR_T1-Flair)	0.33	1.00	0.33	1.00
2 (CT/MR_T2)	0.33	1.00	0	0.00
3 (CT/MR_T1-Flair)	0	0.00	0	0.00
4 (CT/MR_T1-Gd)	0.67	2.00	0	0.00
5 (CT/MR_T1-Gd)	-	-	-	-
6 (CT/MR_T1-3D)	0.33	1.00	0	0.00
7 (CT/MR_T1-Flair)	0	0.00	0.33	1.00
8 (CT/MR_T1-Gd)	0	0.00	0.33	1.00
9 (CT/MR_T2)	0	0.00	0.33	1.00
10(CT/MR_T1-Flair)	0	0.00	0	0.00
11(CT/MR_T1-3D)	0	0.00	0	0.00
12(CT/MR_T1-Flair)	-	-	-	-
13(CT/MR_T1-Gd)	0	0.00	0	0.00
14(CT/MR_T1-Gd)	0	1.41	0	0.00
Ave ($\Sigma\|\delta\|/N$)	0.1	0.5	0.1	0.3
Std Dev (σ)	0.3	0.7	0.3	0.5

Table 3. Misalignment of the MMI-based automatic registration, corrected by the 3DVIR. (taken from Li, et al, IJROBP, 2005, with permission)

These comparison results indicate that the 3DVIR is superior to the 2D visual fusion method in both accuracy and performance (about 5-times faster). Majority (93%) of the 2D fusion results carries registration errors that are hinden from the observer. Similarly, the MMI auto-registration results have smaller errors and the 3DVIR is sensitive enough to detect them. Two disadvantages are found in the 3DVIR: (1) only rigid anatomy can be used as registration landmarks, and (2) the 3DVIR cannot be used by colour-blind observer. These can be resolved by using deformable transformation and quantitative criterion in the future.

4. Clinical Applications of Volumetric Image Registration

4.1 Multi-modality Image-based Radiotherapy Treatment Planning

In radiation therapy, multi-modality images, such as CT, MRI and PET, are increasingly applied in the treatment planning system for more accurate target delineation and target localization (Nestle, et al, 2009). When these imaging modalities are used, the bony anatomy, soft tissue, as well as tumour metabolic/physiologic features are included to provide a comprehensive view of the treatment target and surrounding normal tissues. Image registration is a critical process to align these imaging features in space and in time for treatment planning (Schad et al, 1987, Pelizzari, et al, 1989, Low, et al, 2003, Vedam, et al, 2003, Keall, et al, 2004, Xie, et al, 2004, Li, et al, 2005, Citrin, et al, 2005, Wolthaus, et al, 2005).

With high accuracy of the 3DVIR, target delineation and localization should be improved for the gross tumour volume (GTV) determination at the beginning of treatment planning. Clinically, microscopic extension of the lesion (GTV) is also considered part of the treatment target, forming the clinical tumour volume (CTV). Between the treatment plan and delivery, inter-fractional patient setup uncertainty and intra-fractional organ motion uncertainty are included by using a safety margin, forming the planning tumour volume (PTV), in order to have conformal radiation dose to the target (Song & Li, 2008). The accuracy of the target delineation and localization depends on the accuracy of multi-modality image registration. If a registration error is present but unrealized, it could result in cold spot (under-dose) in the target but hot spot in critical structures (over-dose), leading to sub-optimal local tumour control. Therefore, the high accuracy of multimodality image registration is essential for high precision radiation therapy, including intra-/extra-cranial stereotactic radiosurgery or radiotherapy, and the 3DVIR should be useful in radiation therapy planning and delivery.

It is worthwhile to emphasize that visual verification is required and manual adjustment is often necessary. The use of 3DVIR with sub-mm accuracy should preserve or even improve both the accuracy and reliability of automatic image registration, rather than sacrificing accuracy to gain reliability as in the case of 2D visual verification. Because the 2D visual fusion is so widely used in the clinic, the adoption of the 3D alternative to this technique would have significant impacts to the current and future clinical practice.

4.2 Realigning "Co-registered" PET/CT Images

The hybrid PET/CT scanner has been available for a decade (Beyer, et al, 2000), and upon its acceptance by radiological diagnostic and therapeutic clinics, other hybrid scanners, such as SPECT/CT (Bybel, et al, 2008, Chowdhury & Scarsbrook, 2008) and PET/MRI (Pichler, et al, 2008), have also become available. Only hybrid PET/CT scanners are manufactured in the world since 2003, because "co-registered" biological and anatomical images are produced (Townsend, 2008). Such dramatic market change reflects the importance as well as the difficulty of the registration of a biological image to an anatomical image.

The fundamental assumption for the hybrid scanner to work is a motion-less patient during the time frame of the image acquisitions. Therefore, the fixed spatial relationship between the dual scanners can be corrected to produce "co-registration" of the dual images. The CT imaging takes a few seconds, while PET takes 5 to 30 minutes, depending upon the field of view (or region of interest). A head PET imaging takes 5-10 minutes (1-2 bed positions) while the whole-body PET takes 30 minutes (up to 6-bed positions). Thus, the assumption of motion-free patient is only a rough approximation. Although motion correction has been studied through 4D imaging (Li, et al, 2008a), it has not been adopted as a commonly accepted clinical procedure, concerning clinical gain over the cost (including clinical time). Thus, it remains clinically acceptable to use the PET/CT images as "co-registered" images, knowing the presence of misalignment. However, high-precision radiation therapy, such as intra-cranial stereotactic radiosurgery (SRS), requires the overall uncertainty of < ±1.0 mm in target localization. So, the assumption (or approximation) of motion-less patient needs to be re-examined, in order to meet the clinical requirement. One of the approaches reported is to use a MRI-compatible, stereotactic head frame (external fiducials) for PET/CT and MRI imaging, so that their co-registration is guaranteed (Picozzi, et al, 2005). The invasive fixation of the head to the stereotactic frame, which is immobilized to the imaging couch, ensures no head motion during the image acquisition. Therefore, the alignment of the head frame produces highly accurate image registration. However, it is not generally feasible in the clinic for prescribing and scheduling both new PET/CT and new MRI, while the frame is invasively mounted on a patient's skull for SRS treatment in the same day.

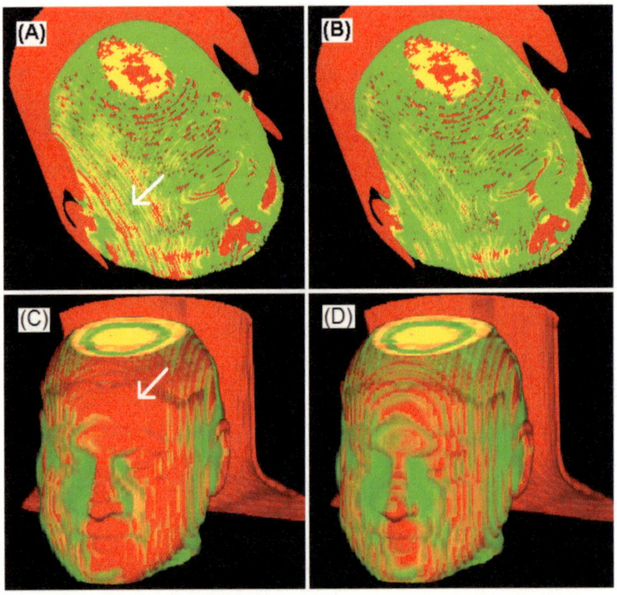

Fig. 10. Correction of misalignments in two "co-registered" PET/CT images: before (A & C) and after (B & D) realignment using the 3DVIR. The arrows point colour inhomogeneity. (taken from Li, et al, IEEE-ISBI, 2007, with permission)

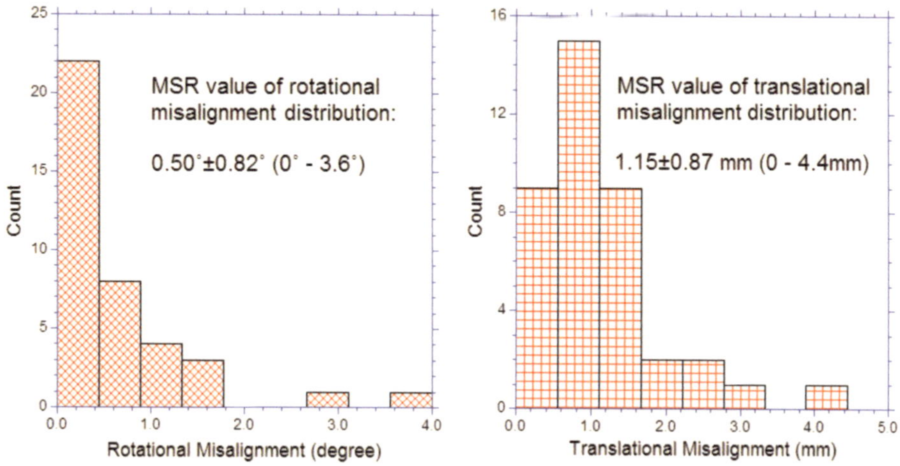

Fig. 11. Rotational and translational misalignments in "co-registered" PET/CT images.

Using the 3DVIR, it is achievable to register PET/CT and MRI images at sub-mm accuracy, as discussed above. Here, we focus on examination and correction of the misalignment in the "co-registered" PET/CT images due to head motion. Thirty-nine patients' cranial images are studied, and about 90% of the patients moved their head during the lengthy PET image acquisition, even with a head immobilization device (a U-shaped frame with ~1 inch foam padding) that is usually used in the nuclear medicine clinic. Among the 39 images, 14 of them are taken from whole-body PET/CT scans, where the time interval between the CT and PET head scans is 30 minutes. As expected, the longer the acquisition time, the greater the movement. Fig. 10 shows the misalignments in a couple of PET/CT images with slightly different head holding devices, and Fig. 11 shows the motion distribution among the 39 patients. The motion results are similar to those detected by infrared camera with a similar head holder (Beyer, et al, 2005). In contrast, the 2D visual fusion technique is not capable of correcting the PET/CT misalignment.

4.3 High Precision Image-guided Radiotherapy Patient Setup

The anatomical deformation and/or change in registration images deteriote the quality of image registration. In image-guided radiotherapy (IGRT), daily patient CT images in the treatment room are acquired to align with the planning CT, reducing the setup uncertainty to ±3 mm from ±5 mm, which was achieved with skin marks and laser alignment. The improved accuracy reduces the safety margin and so increases normal tissue sparing. This is critical to hypo-fractional stereotactic body radiation therapy (SBRT), in which about 5-10 times more radiation dose per fraction than conventional radiotherapy is used, achieving a local control rate as high as 80-90% in early-stage lung cancer patients, similar to surgery (Baumann, et al, 2008, Ball, 2008). The high-precision IGRT daily setup, together with motion control, facilitates SBRT with reduced normal tissue toxicity, permitting escalated dose to the target. Therefore, it is important to gain improved accuracy and reproducibility in target localization through the high precision IGRT patient setup procedure.

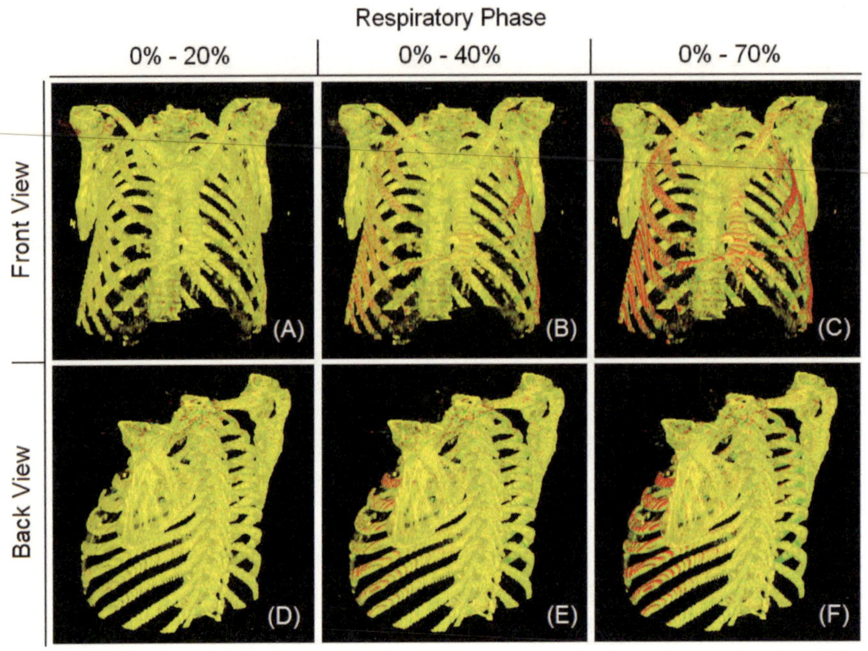

Fig. 12. Identification of motion-free bony landmarks based on 4DCT using the 3DVIR. The respiratory motion causes some bones to move, but not the spine and posterior ribs.

The major uncertainty in registration of thoracic or abdominal images is from respiratory motion and deformation of a patient's anatomy, which varies intra-fractionally and inter-fractionally. So, rigid image registration techniques would produce sub-optimal solution. Although deformable image registration can adapt to the anatomical change, the result cannot be easily utilized in the IGRT setup, since all adjustable machine parameters (3 translational and 1-3 rotational) are related to rigid transformation. Therefore, deformable image registration does not help, while rigid image registration seems reaching its limits.

Patient setup can be separated into two steps: (1) bony landmark alignment and (2) target localization in reference to the bony landmarks (Jiang, 2006). Voluntary or involuntary movements can cause not only the soft tissue but also the bony anatomy to move. Using 4DCT, we have identified the stable (or motion-free) bony anatomy, which are the spine, posterior ribs and clavicles, as shown in Fig. 12. The scapulae are excluded since they are likely to be in different position between daily setups. When a patient lays in supine position on the CT simulation couch or RT treatment couch, these stable bones are most reliable anatomical landmarks for image registration. Therefore, using the motion-free bony landmarks, the accuracy and reproducibility of the IGRT patient setup can be improved.

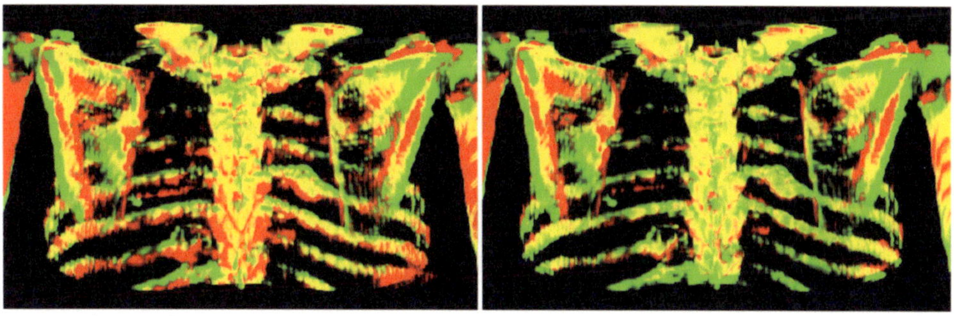

Fig. 13. Before (left) and after (right) the 3DVIR alignment using the stable bony landmarks (the spine, posterior ribs and clavicles). Auto-registration is done for initial alignment (left) .

The on-site CT in the treatment room is usually either kilovoltage cone-beam CT (kV-CBCT), megavoltage CBCT (MV-CBCT), or megavoltage helical CT (MVCT). These CT images usually have lower image quality, in comparison with the simulation CT image, because (1) different imaging configuration and image reconstruction, (2) patient motion during the longer acquisition time (~60 seconds), and/or (3) different photon-tissue interactions due to different beam energies. But, using the 3DVIR technique, which is insensitive to the image quality, the registration of the stable bony anatomy produces a sub-mm accuracy, and the IGRT setup accuracy and reproducibility are consequently improved. In our study, MMI auatomatic registration with a bone density filter is performed first, and the result is adjusted using the 3DVIR, as shown in Fig. 13. It is an on-going study to characterize the target motion within the stable bony coordinate system, so that the 2-step IGRT patient setup procedure can be achieved for a clinical test.

5. Future Directions of Volumetric Image Registration

Clinical research on image registration will continue to meet the challenges from increasing biomedical imaging modalities employed and from higher clinical requirements in terms of precision, automation and deformation. The search of new markers for molecular imaging has dramatically increased, yielding new probes to various biological events (Rajendran, et al, 2006, Nestle, et al, 2009). It promises to depict cancerous activity with high specificity beyond the anatomical GTV or tumour heterogeneity within the morphological change. This will help clinicians for early diagnosis of lesion, for precise delineation of therapeutic target for treatment, or for characterization of tumour microenvironment, including the radio-resistant region within the delineated GTV. One of the examples is probing tumour hypoxic region, which is known to be radio-resistant, and therefore more dose could be prescribed to the hypoxic region within the target volume (Rajendran, et al, 2006). Owing to the modality-insensitive nature and four-concurrent-image capacity, the 3DVIR technique is promising to meet the challenge of increasing use of imaging modalities.

It has been a research forefront to combine image registration with image segmentation, although most research focus on using deformable image registration to assist adaptive segmentation (or active contouring) (Vernuri, et al, 2003, Barder & Hose, 2005, Shekhar, et al, 2007, Wang, et al, 2008). The foundation of the hybrid approach to use segmentation to assist registration is that extracted information from images has higher reliability and more information than the raw data (voxels) in the images. Therefore, a hybridized technique has potential advantages. An early example is Chamfer matching (Borgefors, 1988, van Herk & Kooy, 1994). The 3DVIR is a registration technique hybridized with image classification and visualization. The visually classified anatomic landmark used in the 3DVIR (such as skin and bones) is adjustable volumetric surface that commonly appears in different imaging modalities. Future development toward automation will realize the full potentials of the 3DVIR in multi-modality image registration.

Deformable image registration has recently been revisited with advances of computing power, as well as the challenges in both diagnostic and therapeutic radiological clinics, where patient's motion and deformation have become a clinically relevant issue. Both naturally-occurred (involuntary or voluntary) motion and artificially-induced (surgical or implanting) motion cause anatomical changes and target relocation in external beam radiotherapy and brachytherapy. Significant improvement in performance has been reported using parallel computing technology (Samant, et al, 2008). Once the time comes, suitable algorithm of deformable image registration can be readily introduced into the 3DVIR technique, where image registration transformation and optimization are separated from classification and visualization. So, an automatic deformable 3DVIR could be possible upon sufficient performance improvement of deformable image registration in the future.

For target localization, an alternative approach to deformable image registration has been proposed to adapt to the motion of the diaphragm by calculating its displacement from a reference position based on external torso volume variation. This is achieved by proposing and validating a volume conservation hypothesis within torso (Li, et al, 2009a) and an expandable "piston" respiratory model during quiet respiration (Li, et al, 2009b). Further investigation is required to translate the diaphragm motion into the target motion away from the diaphragm. For many clinical challenges, novel volumetric approaches, including the 3DVIR technique and the volume conservation approach, have shown promises to overcome the clinical problems from volumetric viewpoint.

6. Summary

In this chapter, the 3D volumetric image registration (3DVIR) technique has been introduced and discussed in lieu of increasing use of multi-modality images in the radiotherapy clinic. The foundations of the volumetric image visualization, classification and registration are discussed in details. One of the most important advantages of the 3DVIR is the high accuracy (±0.1 mm), which has been established from three phantom experiments (CT, MRI and PET/CT). This sub-mm accuracy of registration applies to all imaging modalities, including biological imaging. The 3DVIR has shown its superiority to the conventional 2D visual-based fusion technique, which is the only viable visual registration tool in the current clinic. Several clinical applications of the 3DVIR with sub-mm accuracy are shown, including correction of motion-induced misalignment in "co-registered" PET/CT images for intra-cranial stereotactic treatment planning and high precision IGRT patient setup using motion-free bony landmarks for extra-cranial stereotactic treatment delivery. Future directions of the volumetric image registration of multimodality images are also discussed, including several challenging problems in the current clinic.

7. References

Ball, D. (2008). Stereotactic radiotherapy for nonsmall cell lung cancer. *Curr. Opinion Pulmonary Med.*, Vol. 14, pp. 297-302, ISSN: 1070-5287.

Barder, D. C. & Hose, D. R. (2005). Automatic segmentation of medical images using image registration: diagnostic and simulation applicaitons. *J. Med. Eng. Tech.*, Vol. 29, No. 2, pp. 53-63, ISSN: 0309-1902.

Baumann, P.; Nyman, J.; Hoyer, M.; Gagliardi, G.; Lax, I.; Wennberg, B.; Drugge, N.; Ekberg, L.; Friesland, S.; Johansson, K.-A.; Lund, J.-A.; Morhed, E.; Nilsson, K.; Levin, N.; Paludan, M.; Sederholm, C.; Traberg, A.; Wittgren, L. & Lewensohn, R. (2008). Stereotactic body radiotherapy for medically inoperable patients with stage I non-small cell lung cancer - A first report of toxicity related to COPD/CVD in a non-randomized prospective phase II study. *Radiother. Oncol.*, Vol. 88, pp. 359-367, ISSN: 0167-8140.

Beyer, T.; Tellmann, L.; Nickel, I. & Pietrzyk, U. (2005). On the use of positioning aids to reduce misregistration in the head and neck in whole-body PET/CT studies. *J. Nucl. Med.*, Vol. 46, No. 4, pp. 596-602, ISSN: 0161-5505.

Beyer, T.; Townsend, D. W.; Brun, T.; Kinahan, P. E.; Charron, M.; Roddy, R.; Israel, J.; Jerin, J.; Young, J.; Byars, L. & Nutt, R. (2000). A combined PET/CT scanner for clinical oncology. *J. Nucl. Med.*, Vol. 41, pp. 1369-79, ISSN: 0161-5505.

Borgefors, G. (1988). Hierarchical chamfer matching : a parametric edge matching algorithm, *IEEE Trans. Pattern Anal. Machine Intell.*, Vol. 10, pp. 849-865, ISSN: 0162-8828.

Bybel, B.; Brunken, R. C.; DiFilippo, F. P. ; Neumann, D. R. ; Wu, G. & Cerqueira, M. D. (2008). SPECT/CT imaging : clinical utility of an emerging technology. *Radiographics*, Vol. 28, No. 4, pp. 1097-1113, ISSN: 0271-5333.

Chen, C.; Pelizzari, C. A.; Chen, G. T. Y.; Cooper, M. D. & Levin, D. N. (1987). Image analysis of PET data with the aid of CT and MR images. In *Information Processing in Medical Imaging*, C.N. de Graaf & M. A. Viergever (Eds), pp. 601–611. Plenum Press, 1988. ISBN: 0306428075, New York.

Chen, G. T. Y. & Pelizzari, C. A. (1989). Image correlation techniques in radiation therapy planning. *Comput. Med. Imag. Graphics*, Vol. 13, pp. 235–240, ISSN: 0895-6111.

Cho, Z.-H.; Son, Y.-D.; Kim, H.-K.; Kim, K.-N.; Oh, S.-H.; Han, J.-Y.; Hong, I.-K. & Kim, Y.-B. (2007). A hybrid PET-MRI: an integrated molecular-genetic imaging system with HRRT-PET and 7.0-T MRI. *Int. J. Imag. Syst. Tech.*, Vol. 17, No. 4, pp. 252-265, ISSN: 0899-9457.

Chowdhury, F. U. & Scarsbrook, A. F. (2008). The role of hybrid SPECT-CT in oncology: Current and emerging clinical applications. *Clin. Radiol.*, Vol. 63, pp. 241-251, ISSN: 0009-9260.

Citrin, D.; Ning, H.; Guion, P.; Li, G.; Susil, R. C.; Miller, R. W.; Lessard, E.; Pouliot, J.; Xie, H. ; Capala, J. ; Coleman, C. N. ; Camphausen, K. & Menard, C. (2005). Inverse treatment planning based on MRI for HDR prostate brachytherapy, *Int. J. Radiat. Oncol. Biol. Phys.*, Vol. 61, No. 4, pp. 1267-1275, ISSN: 0360-3016.

Cormack, A. M. (1963). Representation of a function by its line integrals, with some radiological applications. *J. Appl. Phys.*, Vol. 34, pp. 2722-2727, ISSN: 0021-8979.

Elhendy, A.; Bax, J. J. & Poldermans, D. (2002). Dobutamine stress myocardial perfusion imaging in coronary artery disease. *J. Nucl. Med.*, Vol. 43, pp. 1634-1646, ISSN: 0161-5505.

Fitzpatrick, J.M.; Hill, D.L.G.; Shyr, Y.; West, J.; Studholme, C. & Maurer, C. R. J. (1998). Visual assessment of the accuracy of retrospective registration of MR and CT images of the brain. *IEEE Trans. Med. Imaging*, Vol. 17, No. 4, pp. 571-585, ISSN: 0278-0062.

Garroway, A. N., Grannell, P. K. & Mansfield, P. (1974). Image formation in NMR by a selective irradiative process. *J. Phys. C: Solid State Phys.*, Vol. 7, L457-L462, ISSN: 0953-8984.

Goldberg, D. E. (1989). *Genetic algorithm in search, optimization and machine learning*, Kluwer Academic Publishers, ISBN: 0-201-15767-5, Boston, MA.

Hibbard, L. S.; McGlone, J. S.; Davis, D. W. & Hawkins, R. A. (1987). Three-dimensional representation and analysis of brain energy metabolism. *Science*, Vol. 236, No. 4809, pp. 1641-1646, ISSN: 0036-8075.

Hibbard, L. S. & Hawkins, R. A. (1988). Objective image alignment for three-dimensional reconstruction of digital autoradiograms. *J. Neurosci. Methods*, Vol. 26, pp. 55-74, ISSN: 0165-0270.

Hill, D. L.; Batchelor, P. G.; Holden, M. & Hawkes, D. J. (2001). Medical image registration. *Phys. Med. Biol.*, Vol. 46, pp. R1-R45, ISSN: 0031-9155.

Hounsfield, G. N. (1973). Computerized transverse axial scanning (tomography). 1. Description of system, *Br. J. Radiol.*, Vol. 46, No. 552, pp. 1016-1022, ISSN: 0007-1285.

Jaffray, D.; Kupelian, P.; Djemil, T. & Macklis, R. M. (2007). Review of image-guided radiation therapy. *Expert. Rev. Anticancer. Ther.*, Vol. 7, pp. 89-103, ISSN: 1473-7140.

Jiang, S. B. (2006). Technical aspects of image-guided respiration-gated radiation therapy. *Med. Dosim.*, Vol. 31, No. 2, pp. 141-151, ISSN: 0958-3947.

Keall, P. (2004). 4-dimesional computed tomography imaging and treatment planning. *Semin. Radiat. Oncol.*, Vol. 14, pp. 81-90, ISSN: 1053-4296.

Kirkpatrick, S.; Gelatt, C. D. & Vecchi, M. P. (1983). Optimization by simulated annealing. *Science*, Vol. 220, No. 4598, pp. 671-680, ISSN: 0036-8075.

Lauterbur, P. C. (1973). Image formation by induced local interactions: examples employing nuclear magnetic resonance. *Nature*, Vol. 242 (March), pp. 190-191, ISSN: 0028-0836.

Li, G.; Xie, H.; Ning, H.; Capala, J.; Arora, B. C.; Coleman, C. N.; Camphausen, K. & Miller, R. W. (2005). A novel 3D volumetric voxel registration technique for volume-view-guided image registration of multiple imaging modalities. *Int. J. Radiat. Oncol. Biol. Phys.*, Vol. 63, No. 1, pp. 261-273, ISSN: 0360-3016.

Li, G.; Xie, H.; Ning, H.; Citrin, D.; Capala, J.; Maass-Moreno, R.; Coleman, C. N.; Camphausen, K. & Miller, R. W. (2007). Registering molecular imaging information into anatomic images with improved spatial accuracy. *Proceedings of IEEE Int. Symp. Biomed. Imaging*, pp. 1144-1147, ISBN: 1-4244-0672-2, Arlington, VA, April 12-15, 2007.

Li, G.; Citrin, D.; Camphausen, K.; Mueller, B. ; Burman, C. ; Mychalczak, B. ; Miller, R. W. & Song, Y. (2008a). Advances in 4D Medical Imaging and 4D radiation therapy. *Technol. Cancer Res. Treat.*, Vol. 7, No. 1 (Feb.), pp. 67-81, ISSN: 1533-0346.

Li, G.; Citrin, D.; Miller, R. W.; Camphausen, K.; Mueller, B.; Mychalczak, B. & Song, Y. (2008b). 3D and 4D medical image registration combined with image segmentation and visualization. In: *Encyclopedia of Healthcare Information Systems*, Wickramasinghe, N. & Geisler, E. (Eds.), pp. 1-9, IGI Global, ISBN: 978-1-59904-889-5, Hershey, PA.

Li, G.; Xie, H.; Ning, H.; Citrin, D.; Capala, J.; Maass-Moreno, R.; Guion, P.; Arora, B.; Coleman, N.; Camphausen, K. & Miller, R. W. (2008c). Accuracy of 3D volumetric image registration based on CT, MR and PET/CT phantom experiments. *J. Appl. Clin. Med. Phys.*, Vol. 9, No. 4, pp. 17-36, ISSN: 1526-9914.

Li, G.; Arora, N.; Xie, H.; Ning, H.; Lu, W.; Low, D.; Citrin, D.; Kaushal, A.; Zach, L.; Camphausen, K. & Miller R. W. (2009a). Quantitative prediction of respiratory tidal volume based on the external torso volume change: a potential volumetric surrogate. *Phys. Med. Biol.*, Vol. 54, pp. 1963-1978, ISSN: 0031-9155.

Li, G.; Xie, H.; Ning, H.; Lu, W.; Low, D.; Citrin, D.; Kaushal, A.; Zach, L.; Camphausen, K. & Miller R. W. (2009b). A novel analytical approach to predict respiratory diaphragm motion based on torso volume variation. *Phys. Med. Biol.*, Vol. 54, pp. 4113-4130, ISSN: 0031-9155.

Ling, C. F.; Humm, J.; Larson, S.; Amols, H.; Fuks, Z.; Leivel, S. & Koutcher, J. A. (2000). Towards multidimensional radiation therapy (MDCRT): Biological imaging and biological conformality. *Int. J. Radiat. Oncol. Biol. Phys.*, Vol. 47, pp. 551-560, ISSN: 0360-3016.

Low, D. A.; Nystrom, M.; Kalinin, E.; Parikh, P.; Dempsey, J. F.; Bradley, J. D.; Mutic, S.; Wahab, S. H.; Islam, T.; Christensen, G.; Politte, D. G. & Whiting, B. R. (2003). A method for the reconstruction of four-dimensional synchronized CT scans acquired during free breathing. *Med. Phys.*, Vol. 30, pp. 1254-1263, ISSN: 0094-2405.

Maintz, J.B.A. & Viergever, M.A. (1998). A survey of medical image registration. *Med. Image Anal.*, Vol. 2, No. 1, pp. 1-36, ISSN: 1361-8415.

Mansfield, P. & Maudsley, A. A. (1977). Medical imaging by NMR. *Br. J. Radiol.*, Vol. 50, No. 591, pp. 188-194, ISSN: 0007-2460.

Nestle, U.; Weber, W.; Hentschel, M. & Grosu A.-L. (2009). Biological imaging in radiation therapy: role of positron emission tomography. *Phys. Med. Biol.*, Vol. 54, pp. R1-R25, ISSN: 0031-9155.

Osman, M. M.; Cohade, C.; Nakamoto, Y.; Marshall, L. T.; Leal, J. P. & Wahl, L. W. (2003). Clinically significant inaccurate localization of lesions with PET/CT: frequency in 300 patients. *J. Nucl. Med.*, Vol. 44, pp. 240-243, ISSN: 0161-5505.

Pelizzari, C. A.; Chen, G. T. Y.; Spelbring, D. R.; Weichselbaum, R. R. & Chen, C. T. (1989). Accurate three-dimensional registration of CT, PET and/or MR images of the brain. *J. Comput. Assist. Tomogr.*, Vol. 13, pp. 20–26, ISSN: 0363-8715.

Phelps, M. E.; Hoffman, E. J.; Maulani, N. A. & Ter-Pogossian, M. M. (1975). Application of annihilation coincidence detection to transaxial reconstruction tomography. *J. Nucl. Med.*, Vol. 16, No. 3, pp. 210-224, ISSN: 0161-5505.

Pichler, B. J.; Judenhofer, M. S. & Pfannenberg, C. (2008). Mulimodality imaging approaches: PET/CT and PET/MRI. In: W. Semmler & M. Schwaiger, (Eds.) *Molecular Imaging I*,

Handbook of Experimental Pharmocology, Vol. 185/I, Springer, ISBN: 978-3-540-72717-0, Berlin.

Picozzi, P.; Rizzo, G.; Landoni, C.; Attuati, L.; Franzin, A.; Messa, C.; Ferrari da Passano, C.; Bettinardi, V. & Fazio, F. (2005). A simplified method to integrate metabolic images in stereotactic procedures using a PET/CT scanner. *Stereotact. Funct. Neurosurg.*, Vol. 83, pp. 208-212, ISSN: 1011-6125.

Pluim, J. P. W.; Maintz, J. B. A. & Viergever, M. A. (2003). Mutual-information-based registration of medical images: a survey. *IEEE Trans. Med. Imag*ing, Vol. 22, No. 8 (Aug), pp. 986-1004, ISSN: 0278-0062.

Rajendran, J. G.; Hendrickson, K. R. G.; Spence, A. M.; et al, (2006). Hypoxia imaging-directed radiation treatment planning. *Eur. J. Nucl. Med. Mol. Imag.*, Vol. 33, No. 13, pp. S44-S52, ISSN: 1619-7070.

Samant, S. S.; Xia, J.; Muyan-Ozcelik, P. & Owens, J. D. (2008). High performance computing for deformable image registration: towards a new paradigm in adaptive radiotherapy. *Med. Phys.*, Vol. 35, No. 8, pp. 3546-3553, ISSN: 0094-2405.

Schad, L. R.; Boesecke, R.; Schlegel, W.; Hartmann, G. H.; Sturm, G. H.; Strauss, L. G. & Lorenz, W. J. (1987). Three dimensional image correlation of CT, MR and PET studies in radiotherapy treatment of brain tumors. *J. Comp. Assis. Tomogr.*, Vol. 11, pp. 948–954, ISSN: 0363-8715.

Schroeder, W.; Martin, K. & Lorensen, B. (2004). *The visualization toolkit*, 3rd Ed, Kitware, Inc., ISBN: 1-930934-12-2, the USA.

Shekhar, R.; Lei, P.; Castro-Pareja, C. R.; Plishker, W. L. & D'Souza, W. (2007). Automatic segmentation of phase-correlated CT scans through nonrigid image registration using geometrically regularized free-form deformation. *Med. Phys.*, Vol. 34, No. 7, pp. 3054-3066, ISSN: 0094-2405.

Snyman, J. A. (2005). Practical mathematical optimization: an introduction to basic optimization theory and classical and new gradient-based algorithms, Springer Publishing, ISBN: 0-387-24348-8, New York.

Song, Y. & Li, G., (2008). Current and future trends in radiation therapy, In: *Principles and Advanced Methods in Medical Imaging and Image Analysis*, Dhawan, A.P., Huang, H.K. & Kim, D.-K. (Eds), pp.745-781, World Scientific, ISBN: 978-981-270-534-1, New Jersey.

Ter-Pogossian, M. M.; Phelps, M. E. & Hoffman, E. J. (1975). A positron-emission transaxial tomgraph for nuclear imaging (PET). *Radiology*, Vol. 114, No. 1, pp. 89-98, ISSN: 0039-8419.

Toga, A. W. & Banerjee, P. K. (1993). Registration revisited. *J. Neurosci. Methods*, Vol. 48, pp. 1-13, ISSN: 0165-0270.

Townsend, D. W. (2008). Positron emission tomography/computed tomography. *Semin Nucl. Med.*, Vol. 38, pp.152–166, ISSN: 0001-2998.

Vaarkamp, J. (2001). Reproducibility of interactive registration of 3D CT and MR pediatric treatment planning head images. *J. Appl. Clin. Med. Phys.*, Vol. 2, pp. 131–137, ISSN: 1526-9914.

van Herk M. & Kooy H.M. (1994). Automatic three-dimensional correlation of CT-CT, CT-MRI, and CT-SPECT using chamfer matching. *Med. Phys.*, Vol. 21, pp. 1163–1178, ISSN: 0094-2405.

Vedam, S. S.; Keall, P. J.; Kini, V. R.; Mostafavi, H.; Shikla, H. P. & Mohan, R. (2003). Acquiring a four-dimensional computed tomography dataset using an external respiratory signal. *Phys. Med. Biol.*, Vol. 48, pp. 45-62, ISSN: 0031-9155.

Venot, A.; Lebruchec, J. F. & Roucayrol, J. C. (1984). A new class of similarity measures for robust image registration. *Comp. Vision, Graphics Image Processing,* Vol. 28, pp. 176–184, ISSN: 0734-189X.

Vernuri, B. C.; Ye, J.; Chen, Y. & Leonard, C. M. (2003). Image registration via level-set motion: Applications to atlas-based segmentation. *Med. Image Anal.*, Vol. 7, pp. 1-20, ISSN: 1361-8415.

Viola, P. & Wells, III, W.M. (1995). Alignment by maximization of mutual information. *Proceedings of Int. Conf. Computer Vision,* pp. 16-23, ISBN: 0-8186-7042-8, Boston, MA, June 20-23, IEEE Computer Society Press, Los Alamitos, CA.

Wang, H.; Garden, A. S.; Zhang, L.; Wei, X.; Ahamad, A.; Kuban, D. A.; Komaki, R.; O'Daniel, J.; Zhang, Y.; Mohan, R. & Dong, L. (2008). Performance evaluation of automatic anatomy segmentation algorithm on repeat or four-dimensional computed tomography images using deformable image registration method. *Int. J. Radiat. Oncol. Biol. Phys.*, Vol. 71, No. 1, pp. 210-219, ISSN: 0360-3016.

West, J.; Fitzpartick J.M.; Wang M.Y.; Dawant, B. M.; Maurer, C. R. Jr.; Kessler, R. M.; Maciunas, R. J.; Barillot, C.; Lemoine, D.; Collignon, A.; Maes, F.; Suetens, P.; Vandermeulen, D.; van den Elsen, P. A.; Napel, S.; Sumanaweera, T. S.; Harkness, B.; Hemler, P. F.; Hill, D. L. G.; Hawkes, D. J.; Studholme, C. ; Maintz, J. B. A.; Viergever, M. A.; Malandain, G.; Pennec, X.; Noz, M. E.; Maguire, G. Q. Jr.; Pollack, M. C.; Pelizzari, A.; Robb, R. A.; Hanson, D. & Woods, R. P. (1997). Comparison and evaluation of retrospective intermodality brain image registration techniques. *J. Comput. Assist. Tomogr.*, Vol. 21, No.4, pp.554-568, ISSN: 0363-8715.

Wolthaus, J. W. H.; van Herk, M.; Muller, S. H.; Belderbos, J. S. A.; Lebesque, J. V.; de Bois, J. A.; Rossi, M. M. G. & Damen, E. M. F. (2005). Fusion of respiration-correlated PET and CT scans: correlated lung tumor motion in anatomical and functional scans. *Phys. Med. Biol.*, Vol. 50, pp. 1569-1583, ISSN: 0031-9155.

Xie, H.; Li, G.; Ning, H.; Menard, C.; Coleman, C. N. & Miller, R. W. (2004). 3D voxel fusion of multi-modality medical images in clinic treatment planning system. *Proceedings of IEEE Computer-Based Medical Systems,* pp. 40-46, ISBN: 0-7695-2104-5, Bethesda, MD, June, IEEE Computer Society Press, Los Alamitos, CA.

2

Full Range Swept-Source Optical Coherence Tomography with Ultra Small Fiber Probes for Biomedical Imaging

Youxin Mao, Costel Flueraru and Shoude Chang
Institute for Microstructural Sciences, National Research Council Canada
1200 Montreal Rd, Ottawa, K1A 0R6, ON, Canada

1. Introduction

Optical coherence tomography (OCT) (Huang et al., 1991) is becoming an increasingly important imaging tool for many applications in biology and medicine, such as diagnosis and guided surgery. Due to its high resolution and fiber catheter capability, OCT is more attractive than current imaging technologies, such as ultrasound. An OCT system with higher sensitivity is essentially important for imaging the biomedical turbid tissue because the backscattered optical signal from the tissue is extremely weak. In the earlier stages of OCT imaging, axial (depth) ranging is provided by linearly scanned low-coherence interferometry (Youngquist et al., 1987; Takada et al., 1987). This method of OCT, referred to as time-domain OCT (TD-OCT), has a relatively slow sensitivity and imaging speed because its sensitivity is inversely proportional to the imaging speed. Fourier domain techniques in OCT have received much attention in recent years due to its significant sensitivity and speed advantages over TD-OCT (Leitgeb et al., 2003; [a]Choma et al., 2003; De Boer et al., 2003). Fourier domain methods include spectral-domain OCT (SD-OCT) and swept-source OCT (SS-OCT). In SD-OCT, individual spectral components of low coherence light are detected separately by the use of a spectrometer and a charge-coupled device (CCD) array (Fercher et al., 1995; Hausler & Lindner, 1998) CCD arrays however may introduce phase washout problems during the pixel integration time. Furthermore, detection using a spectrometer and CCD array cannot implement differential optical detection. SS-OCT uses a wavelength-swept laser source and photodetectors based on optical frequency-domain reflectometry for imaging (Chinn et al., 1997; [a]Yun et al., 2003). SS-OCT is particularly important for imaging in the 1.3 μm wavelength range, where low-cost detector arrays are not available. The larger penetration depth of the OCT image by using the 1.3 μm wavelength light source is important for the biomedical turbid tissues, such as human skin and arterial plaque, in comparison to that by using 1.0 μm or shorter wavelength light source. SS-OCT could also make possible for a quadrature interferometry based on multi-port fiber couplers, for example, 3x3 quadrature interferometer ([b]Choma et al., 2003; [a]Mao et al., 2008). Due to its ability to have instantaneous complex signals with stable phase information, OCT with a 3x3 quadrature interferometer could suppress the complex conjugate artifact naturally, therefore to double the effective imaging depth. By detection of the phase from the complex signals, it also could exploit additional information of the tissue to enhance image contrast, obtain functional information, and perform quantitative measurements (Sticker et al., 2001; [a]Zhao et la. 2000). In addition, SS-OCT could make possible for an unbalanced input fiber interferometer and differential output detection by using a Mach-Zehnder interferometer. The unbalanced input could emit larger portion of the optical power from optical source to the tissue than that to the reference mirror for increasing sensitivity (Rollins & Izatt, 1999). The differential detection is used to reduce the excess intensity noise to further sensitivity enhancement compared to SD-OCT (Podoleanu, 2000).

In SS-OCT, the location of a scatterer within tissue is obtained by a Fourier transformation of the optical measurement. When the real component of the interferometric signal is the only detected part, a complex conjugate artifact is introduced after the Fourier transformation. This artifact prevents the distinction between positive and negative object depths thereby reducing the effective imaging range by half. As imaging range is important in biomedical applications, methods for removing this complex conjugate artifact to achieve full range in SS-OCT are of significant interest. Different full-range SS-OCT imaging methods which measure the complex component of the interferometric signal by shifting the phase of the reference and/or sample reflections have been reported. This phase shift has been implemented by a high-speed electronic-optical phase modulator (Zhang et al., 2004), two high-speed acoustic-optical frequency shifters (Yun et al., 2004), and a pair of linearly polarized beams (Vakoc et al., 2006). All of these methods suffered from significant image corruption resulting from any small variations in the phase shift or birefringence of used materials. Recently, acquisition of both real and imaginary interferometric components was demonstrated using Michelson quadrature interferometers using 3x3 fused fiber couplers and non-differential optical detection (Choma et al., 2003; Sarunic et al., 2005; Sarunic et al., 2006). In reference (Sarunic et al., 2005), a 3x3 Michelson quadrature interferometer with balanced differential detection was used for acquiring the complex interferometric signal. Signal attenuation was used to achieve such balanced differential detection which resulted in loss of optical power. In this system, there was a non-complementary phase shift of 60° between the two output interferometric signals that needed to be converted to quadrature components by a trigonometric manipulation. In addition, due to the nature of the Michelson interferometer, the optical output power at one of the ports of the 3x3 coupler (1/3 of the source power) was not utilized in these references.

A wavelength-swept laser source with high-speed, high power, long coherence, i.e. narrow instantaneous linewidth, and wide sweeping range is essential for SS-OCT because the imaging speed, sensitivity, depth and resolution directly rely on the sweeping rate, output power, coherence length and sweeping range of the source. A high powered wavelength-swept laser is also needed for multi-channel SS-OCT. Much progress has been made on the development of high-speed swept lasers, but their output power has been limited. A sweeping repetition rate of 115 kHz has been demonstrated by using a 128-facet polygon scanner (Oh et al., 2005). Because the cavity length in this swept laser is not short enough, the photons do not have sufficient time within the laser cavity to build up the optical power and to narrow the linewidth through mode competition. That is why the resultant optical average power and instantaneous linewidth were low (23 mW) and wide (0.23 nm), respectively. A better result of higher average power of 54 mW (Oh et al., 2008) has been reported, but no description of the laser system has been given. Fourier-domain mode locking (FDML) technique is an alternative approach to achieving higher sweeping speed while a higher optical power is preserved, which was reported recently (Huber et al., 2006a). An FDML wavelength-swept laser with a long cavity has a quasi-stationary operation where one wavelength propagates through the cavity and returns to an optical narrow bandpass filter. Consequently, the laser generates a sequence of narrowband optical wavelength sweeps at the cavity repetition rate. An FDML wavelength swept laser with sweeping repetition up to 370 kHz using a Fabry-Perot tunable filter has been reported (Huber et al., 2006b). Although a narrow (~ 0.1 nm) instantaneous linewidth was reached, the direct output power of this laser was low. To achieve an average output power of 36 mW at the sweeping repetition of 100 kHz, an external semiconductor optical power booster had to be used. However, an amplifier outside the cavity could cause performance degradation, e.g., an increase in linewidth (Huber et al., 2005) and system noise (Rao et al., 2007), thereby reducing the penetration depth and sensitivity of an OCT system.

In the most optically nontransparent tissues, OCT has a typical imaging depth limitation of 1-3 mm. As a result, the earliest *in vivo* OCT imaging of tissue microstructure and microvasculature was restricted to a few transparent or superficial organ sites, such as the retina (Yazdanfar et al., 2000; White et al., 2003) and skin (Zhao et al., 2000). To overcome this depth limitation, optical probes, such as endoscopes, catheters, and needles have been investigated for *in vivo* OCT imaging in mucosal layers of the gastrointestinal tract (Tran et al., 2004; Yang et al., 2005a), deep organs and tissues (Li et al., 2000; Yang et al., 2005b), and inter-arterial and intra-vascular (Fujimoto et al., 1999; Diaz-Sandoval et al., 2005). However, for the imaging of small lumen, narrow space, and deep tissue and organ of humans and small animals, a key concern is the possible damage from the mechanical insertion of the optical probe. Therefore it is critical to develop an ultra-small optical probe that is compatible with the current optical biomedical imaging systems, which results in minimum tissue damage. *In vivo* optical imaging of internal tissues is generally performed using a fiber-optic probe, since an optical fiber can be easily and cheaply produced with a diameter of less than 150 μm. The key components of such optical fiber probe include a small lens and a beam director, where both provide a focused optical beam directing it to a location of interest through a guide-wire. Traditionally, this type of small optical probe has been implemented by attaching a small radial graded refractive index (GRIN) glass rod lens or called SELFOC lens with a size range of 0.25-1.0 mm and a tiny glass micro-prism to a single mode fiber (SMF) with optical adhesive or optical epoxy (Li et al., 2000). However, the gluing of a separate small lens and a tiny prism to a fiber is a complex fabrication process that results in a low quality optical interface. A new probe design that uses optical fiber lenses, e.g., fiber GRIN lens or fiber ball lens, has been proposed (Swanson et al., 2002; Shishkov et al., 2006). The main advantage of fiber lenses over conventional glass lenses are their small size, ability to auto-align to a fiber, thus creating a fusion-spliced interface with low loss, low back-reflection, and high mechanical integrity. In addition, a beam director can be easily attached to the fiber lenses by the fusion-splice of a polished fiber spacer and direct polish on the ball lens. Beam quality of a fiber-optic probe is crucial for the imaging system. Ideal characteristics of a fiber-optic probe include a high Gaussian beam intensity profile, an appropriate intensity-distance shape, high flexibility, and low optical aberration and loss.

Swanson *et al.*and Shishkov *et al.* proposed the fiber based optic probes design, but presented the variations of probe structure instead of the characteristics of their performance (Swanson et al., 2002; Shishkov et al., 2006). Reed *et al.* demonstrated the usage of such probes with emphasis on their insertion loss only (Reed et al., 2002). Yang *et. al.* (Yang et al., 2005b), Jafri *et. al.* (Jafri et al., 2005), and Li *et. al.* (Li et al., 2006) reported OCT images without detailed characterization of the used fiber lens based probes. We recently reported design, fabrication, and characterization of the fiber probes with comparison in detail the actual optical performance of a fiber-based optic probe with modeling results (Mao et al., 2007; Mao et al., 2008).

In the second section in this chapter, we present theoretical and experimental results for a 3x3 Mach-Zehnder quadrature interferometer to acquire a complex interferometric signal for SS-OCT system. We introduce a novel unbalanced differential detection method to improve the overall utilization of optical power and provide simultaneous access to the complementary phase components of the complex interferometric signal. No calculations by trigonometric relationships are needed. We compare the performance for our setup to that of a similar interferometer with a commonly used balanced detection technique. We demonstrate complex conjugate artifact suppression of 27 dB obtained in a swept-source optical coherence tomography using our unbalanced differential detection. We show that our unbalanced differential detection has increased signal-to-noise ratio by at least 4 dB comparing to a commonly used balanced detection technique. In the third section, we demonstrate a Fourier-domain mode-lock (FDML) wavelength-swept laser based on a polygon scanner filter and a high-efficiency semiconductor optical amplifier. Peak and average output powers of 98 mW and 71 mW, respectively, have been achieved without an external amplifier, while the wavelength was swept continuously in a full wavelength of 113 nm at center wavelength of 1303 nm. A unidirectional wavelength sweeping rate of 7452 nm/ms (65.95 kHz repetition rate) was achieved by using a 72 facet polygon with a rotational rate, R, of 916 revolutions per second. The instantaneous linewidth of this laser is 0.09 nm, which corresponds to a coherence length of 16 mm. We also construct an OCT system that uses our laser source where we have shown that its parameters are optimized for this application. In the fourth section, we discuss design methods and fabrication techniques of fiber-lens-based optic probes. We compare in detail measured performance with expected theoretical performance. Finally, we demonstrate the images of human skins, animal arterial plaque and heart tissues acquired from our catheter-based complex SS-OCT, which proves our SS-OCT system with fiber catheter is most suitable for the applications of biomedical imaging.

2. Full Range (Complex) Optical Coherence Tomography System

2.1 Theoretical Analysis of the Complex System

An MZI utilizing a 3x3, two 2x2 fiber couplers, and two differential detectors is shown in Fig. 1. A 90/10 2x2 fiber coupler is used as a power divider of the light source: 90% power to the sample and 10% power to reference arms. This is an advantage of the MZI (Rollins & Izatt, 1999), which allows more light to the sample arm for compensating the lower reflection of a biological sample in an OCT system. The 3x3 fiber coupler serves not only as a combiner of the two signals from the sample and reference arms, but also provides three phase related output interferometric signals. To form two phase related differential detections, which are necessitated to obtain the real and imaginary parts of the interferometric signal, one of the output ports of the 3x3 coupler is split using one 50/50 2x2 fiber coupler. Two differential detectors were constructed by combining one output of the 2x2 coupler and one of the remaining outputs of the 3x3 coupler. We note that the input signals for these differential detectors are not balanced, but no optical power is lost. For comparison, the different unbalanced differential detection methods with different input power ratios, achieved by adjusting two additional fiber attenuators, are also shown in Fig. 1. When the input power ratio is adjusted to achieve balanced detection (i.e. attenuation α = 0.5), the DC component of the interferometric signal could be dynamically removed, but one third of the optical power would be lost.

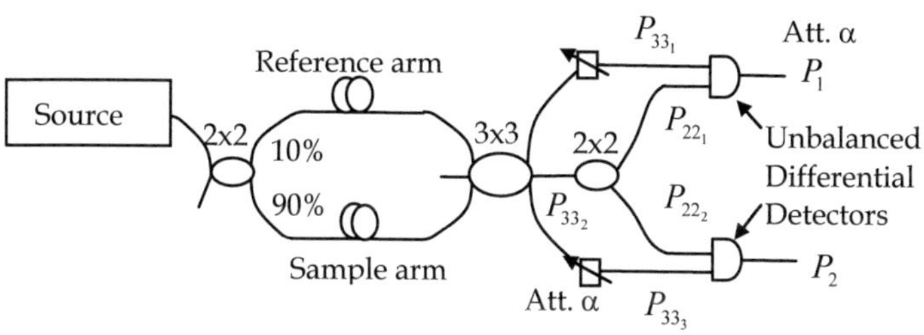

Fig. 1. Mach-Zehnder interferometer using a 3x3 and two 2x2 fiber couplers to form two channel unbalanced (attenuation α = 1 - 0.5) and balanced (attenuation α = 0.5) differential detections for acquiring real and imaginary parts of the interferometric signal.

To analyze our setup we could use transfer matrix descriptions for both 2x2 and 3x3 couplers (Sheem, 1981; Priest, 1982). The output electric field of a 2x2 coupler, $\mathbf{E}_{\mathbf{out}_{2x2}} = [E_{out_1} \quad E_{out_2}]^T$, due to an input electric field, $\mathbf{E}_{\mathbf{in}_{2x2}} = [E_{in_1} \quad E_{in_2}]^T$, where T denotes matrix transposition, is given by $\mathbf{E}_{\mathbf{out}_{2x2}} = \mathbf{M}_{\mathbf{2x2}}\mathbf{E}_{\mathbf{in}_{2x2}}$, where

$$\mathbf{M}_{\mathbf{2x2}_{\mathbf{50/50}}} = \begin{bmatrix} \sqrt{0.5} & -j\sqrt{0.5} \\ -j\sqrt{0.5} & \sqrt{0.5} \end{bmatrix} \tag{1}$$

presents the transfer matrix of a 50/50 2x2 coupler, and

$$\mathbf{M}_{\mathbf{2x2}_{\mathbf{90/10}}} = \begin{bmatrix} \sqrt{0.9} & -j\sqrt{0.1} \\ -j\sqrt{0.1} & \sqrt{0.9} \end{bmatrix} \tag{2}$$

is the transfer matrix of a 90/10 2x2 coupler. Similarly, the output electric field of a 3x3 coupler could be written as $\mathbf{E}_{\mathbf{out}_{3x3}} = \mathbf{M}_{\mathbf{3x3}}\mathbf{E}_{\mathbf{in}_{3x3}}$, where

$$\mathbf{M}_{\mathbf{3x3}} = \frac{e^{-j2K_{cpl}}}{3}\begin{bmatrix} 1 & 1 & 1 \\ 1 & 1 & 1 \\ 1 & 1 & 1 \end{bmatrix} + \frac{e^{j2K_{cpl}}}{3}\begin{bmatrix} 2 & -1 & -1 \\ -1 & 2 & -1 \\ -1 & -1 & 2 \end{bmatrix} \tag{3}$$

and K_{cpl} is the coupling coefficient and equals to 0.7 for a 3x3 coupler with 1/3 power coupling ratio (Sheem, 1981).

The operation of a Mach-Zehnder interferometer could be represented by a cascade of the transfer matrices of the couplers and a matrix representing the phase shift between the sample and reference arms ϕ. Let the input electric field and the matrix representing the phase shift between the sample and reference arms be given by $\mathbf{E_{in}} = [0 \;\; 1 \;\; 0]^T$ and $\mathbf{M_\varphi} = \begin{bmatrix} 0 & 0 & 0 \\ 0 & 1 & 0 \\ 0 & 0 & e^{j\phi} \end{bmatrix}$, respectively. In our setup, the splitter ratio of the first 2x2 coupler is 90/10.

Therefore, the output electric field, $\mathbf{E_{33}(\varphi)} = [E_{33_1}(\phi) \;\; E_{33_2}(\phi) \;\; E_{33_3}(\phi)]^T$ after the 3x3 coupler shown in Fig. 1 is calculated by:

$$\mathbf{E_{33}}(\varphi) = \mathbf{M_{3x3}}\mathbf{M_\varphi}(\phi)\mathbf{M_{2x2_{90/10}}}\mathbf{E_{in}}\,. \tag{4}$$

In the case of the 2x2 coupler after the 3x3 coupler, if the input electric field is given by $\mathbf{E_{in_{2x2}}}(\phi) = [E_{33_2}(\phi) \;\; 0]^T$, the output electric fields, $\mathbf{E_{22_1}}$, $\mathbf{E_{22_2}}$, are obtained by:

$$\mathbf{E_{22_1}}(\phi) = \mathbf{M_{2x2_{50/50}}}\mathbf{E_{in_{2x2}}}(\phi)\,, \tag{5a}$$

$$\mathbf{E_{22_2}}(\phi) = \mathbf{M_{2x2_{50/50}}}\mathbf{E_{in_{2x2}}}(\phi)\,. \tag{5b}$$

Therefore, the related optical powers P_{33_1}, P_{22_1}, P_{22_2}, and P_{33_3} specified in Fig. 1 are calculated by:

$$P \propto \mathbf{E}^*\mathbf{E}\,. \tag{6}$$

The interferometric signal powers P_1 and P_2 from the outputs of the two differential detectors v.s. the attenuation value α and the phase shift between the sample and reference arms ϕ are calculated by subtracting the two optical input signal powers of the detectors, respectively, i.e.,

$$P_1(\phi) = \alpha P_{33_1}(\phi) - P_{22_1}(\phi)\,, \tag{7a}$$

$$P_2(\phi) = \alpha P_{33_3}(\phi) - P_{22_2}(\phi)\,. \tag{7b}$$

The phase differences between the two interferometric signals P_1 and P_2 and the related power levels are obtained by graphing their function curves vs. ϕ.

The real (P_{RE}) and imaginary (P_{IM}) part signals, e.g. quadrature components (0° and 90°), are formed from the interferometric signals P_1 and P_2 acquired at two differential detectors using the following trigonometric equations (Choma et al., 2003):

$$P_{RE}(\phi) = P_1(\phi)\,, \qquad P_{IM}(\phi) = \frac{P_1(\phi)\cos(\Delta\phi) - P_2(\phi)}{\sin(\Delta\phi)} \tag{8}$$

where, $\Delta\phi$ is the phase difference between the interferometric signals P_1 and P_2. The wavelength dependent power splitting ratios of the fiber couplers were neglected in this work for simplicity. SS-OCT A-scans with resolved complex conjugate artifact were obtained by inverse Fourier transformation (IFT) of the complex signal $P_{RE}+jP_{IM}$.

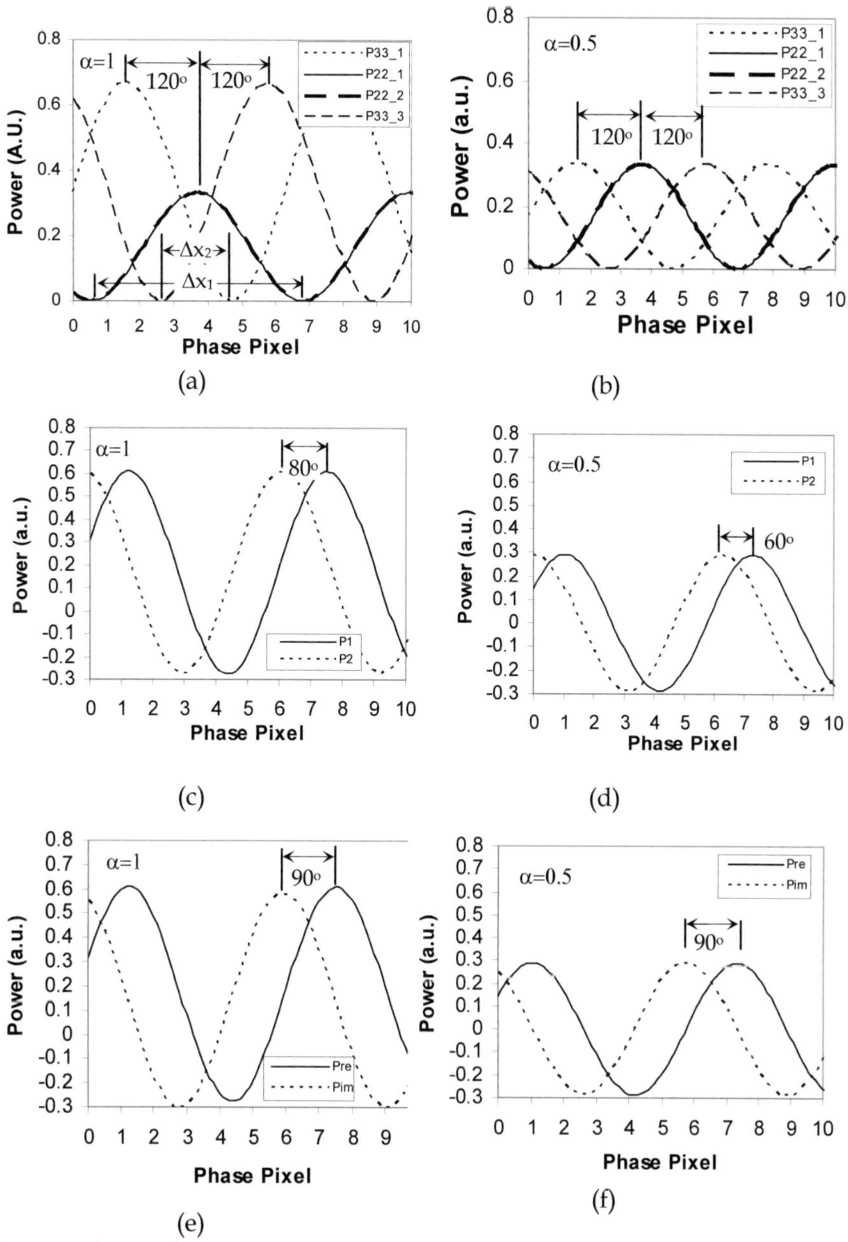

Fig. 2. Theoretical waveforms before (a, b) and after (c, d) the differential detection and after the quadrature signal calculations (e, f) when the attenuation α = 1 (a, c, e) and 0.5 (b, d, f), where α = 1.0 and 0.5 correspond to the unbalanced by a factor of 2 and balanced configurations, respectively.

Fig. 2 shows theoretical waveforms when the attenuation α = 1 (a, c, e) and 0.5 (b, d, f), where α = 1.0 and 0.5 correspond to the unbalanced by a factor of 2 and balanced configurations, respectively. The waveforms shown in Fig.2 (a, b) and (c, d) are calculated before and after the differential detections, respectively, while the waveforms shown in Fig.2 (e, f) are calculated using the Eq. 8. The phase difference Δ was calculated using $\Delta = 2\pi\Delta x_2/\Delta x_1$, where Δx_1 and Δx_2 are the phase pixel intervals of a period and a difference of the two signals, respectively, as illustrated in Fig. 2 (a). The phase differences of 120° between the two input detector signals were obtained for both $\alpha = 0.5$ and 1.0 configurations as shown in Fig. 2 (a, b). This is due to the phase difference resulting from the 3x3 coupler. Because of the power difference of the input signals, the amplitude levels and the phase relationships of the output signals would be different in the two setups as shown in Fig. 2.

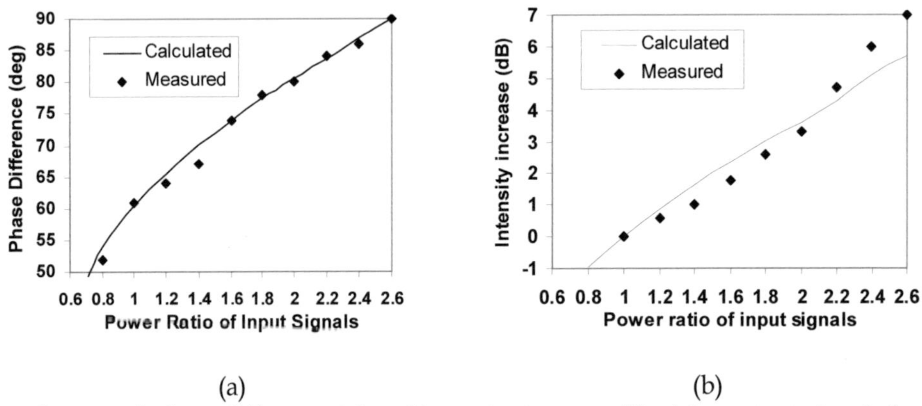

Fig. 3. Theoretical phase difference (a) and intensity increase (b) of the output signals for the unbalanced configuration from the balanced configuration verses power ratio of the two detector input signals, respectively. The experimental results are shown as the points.

Fig. 3 (a) and (b) show theoretical and experimental results of the phase difference and intensity increase of the output signals, P_1 and P_2 for the unbalanced configuration from the balanced configuration versus input power ratios of the detectors, respectively. The phase differences of the output signals are 60° and 80° when power ratios of input signals are 1 (balanced configuration) and 2 (unbalanced configuration), respectively, obtained both in theory and experiment. The intensities of the output signals increase 3dB when the power ratio of input signals is 2 (unbalanced configuration) comparing to the power ratio of input signals is 1 (balanced situation). The input power ratios from 2 to 2.6 for the detectors could be obtained when the coupling ratio of 3x3 was not exactly 1/3. From the results shown in Fig. 3 (a), a 90° phase difference between the detector outputs P_1 and P_2 could be obtained if the input power ratio was 2.6, therefore, no calculations by the trigonometric relationships are needed for obtaining the quadrature signals.

2.2 Method of the Complex OCT System

Fig. 4 shows the experimental setup of the instantaneous complex conjugate resolved swept-source OCT system using the 3x3 Mach-Zehnder interferometer topology with the unbalanced (no attenuators) and balanced (with attenuators) differential detection schemes. The system consisted of a 2x2 single-mode fiber coupler with 90/10 coupling ratio as the input coupler and a 3x3 fiber coupler with coupling ratios of 0.39/0.29/0.32, a 50/50 2x2 fiber couplers and two variable fiber attenuators as the output couplers forming the dual-channel balanced detection.

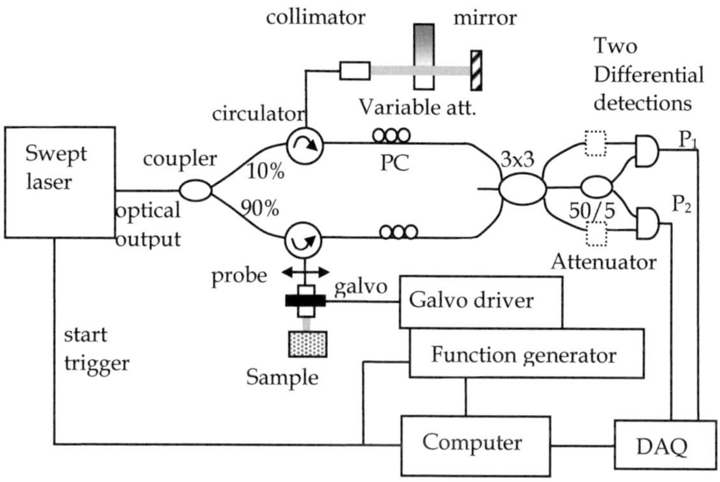

Fig. 4. Schematic diagram of the instantaneous complex conjugate resolved swept-source OCT system using the 3x3 Mach-Zehnder interferometer (MZI) topology with unbalanced (no attenuators) and balanced (with attenuators in the doted line) differential schemes. The coupler ratios of the 3x3 coupler are 0.39/0.29/0.32.

The swept source (HSL2000-HL, Santac) used in the system had a central wavelength of 1320 nm and a full scan wavelength range of 110 nm, which was sweeping linearly with optical frequency with a linearity of 0.2%. The average output power and coherence length of the swept source was 12 mW and 10 mm, respectively. A repetition scan rate of 20 kHz was used in our system and the related duty cycle was 68%. The output light from the swept laser source was launched into the first coupler and then divided into the sample arm with 90% power and reference arm with 10% power by two fiber circulators. The reference arm was arranged with a fiber collimator and a mirror. A variable attenuator was inserted between the collimator and mirror for adjusting the optical power on reference arm to achieve the higher sensitivity. The light was illuminated to a sample through the lensed single mode fiber probe with working distance (focus distance to lens surface in air) of 1.1 mm, depth of field (twice the Rayleigh range in air) of 1.1 mm, and $1/e^2$ spot diameter (transverse resolution) of 27 μm which will be described in the third section in this chapter. A galvanometer (Blue Hill Optical technologies) scanner scanned the fiber probe light transversely on the sample up to 4 mm at 20 Hz with 1000 transverse pixels. The total optical power illuminating on the sample was approximately 10 mW. Two polarization controllers (PC) in both reference and sample arms were used for adjustment to match the polarization state of the two arms. The two-pair output signals from the output couplers were detected with two-pair photodiodes to obtain quadrature signals. Two differential photo-detectors (PDB150C, Thorlabs) were used with adjustable bandwidth. A 3 dB bandwidth of 50 MHz was used in our system. The two detector outputs were digitized using a data acquisition card (DAQ) (PCI 5122, National Instruments) with 14-bit resolution and acquired at a sampling speed of *100 MS/s*. The swept source generated a start trigger signal that was used to initiate the function generator for the galvo scanner and initiate the data acquisition process for each A-scan. Because the swept source was linearly swept with wave-number k, A-scans data with resolved complex conjugate artifact were obtained by a direct inverse Fourier transformation (IFT) from direct DAQ sampling data without any re-sampling process.

2.3 Results and Discussion of Complex OCT system

The performance of the complex conjugate ambiguity resolution in our 3x3 Mach-Zehnder SS-OCT system with the unbalanced configuration could be quantified by comparing the complex conjugate resolved A-scans with the unresolved A-scans. Measurements were taken using a -55dB reflector including coupling loss in the sample arm as shown in Fig. 4. The reference mirror was adjusted to a position such that the difference in optical path length between the two interferometer arms was 500 μm. The extra background noise was subtracted by measuring the reference arm signals with the sample arm blocked.

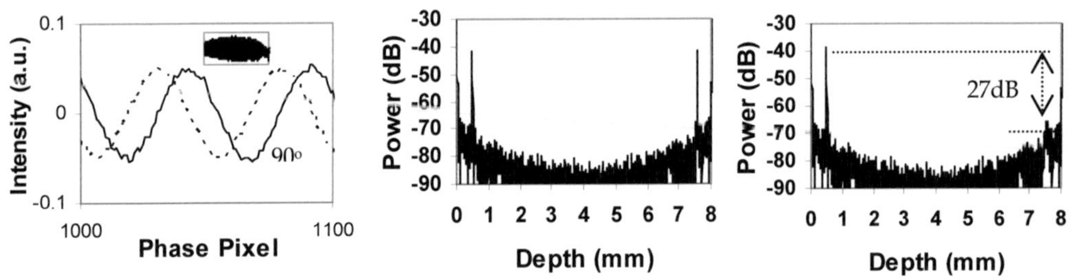

(a) (b) (c)

Fig. 5. The experimental results of the complex conjugate artifact resolution with our 3x3 MZI SS-OCT in the unbalanced differential detection with 3x3 coupler ratio of 0.39/0.29/0.32 in 500 μm path length difference of the sample and reference arms. (a): Measured interferometric signals of the output P_1 and P_2 on two detectors with phase shift of 90°. Inset: Measured full interferometric signals of the output P_1 and P_2. (b): A-scan signals obtained by IFT from a single detector include the complex conjugate artifacts. (c): A-scan signals obtained by IFT directly from the output signals at the two detectors with suppressions of the complex conjugate peaks of 27 dB.

Fig. 5 (a) shows measured waveforms of the output signal P_1 and P_2 from our unbalanced SS-OCT system with 3x3 port configuration as coupler ratio of 0.39/0.29/0.32, i.e., we connected the lowest power port of the 3x3 coupler to the 2x2 coupler. The input power ratios in this unbalanced setup were 2.8 and 2.4 for the two detectors, respectively. We noticed from the full interferometric signals of the output P_1 and P_2 shown in the inset of the Fig. 5 (a) that the DC values of the waveforms in the unbalanced system were removed by the high-pass filter of the detectors. Because a phase difference of 90° between the interferometric signals P_1 and P_2 was obtained, the data of measured P_1 and P_2 was automatically become quadrature signals. Therefore, a minimized complex conjugate artifact was obtained after performing a complex Fourier transform operation directly from the two outputs. Fig. 5 (b) shows the A-scan at 500 μm depth obtained by inverse Fourier transform of a single detector include the complex conjugate artifact. The symmetric reflective peaks were in both positive and negative sides. Fig. 5 (c) shows the complex conjugate resolved A-scan obtained by taking the inverse Fourier transform directly from the output quadrature signals P_1 and P_2. SNR and suppression of the complex conjugate peaks of 52 dB and 27 dB was obtained at about 500 μm depths in our unbalanced differential detection SS-OCT system when the 55dB reflector in the sample arm was used. Therefore, the measured sensitivity of 107 dB was obtained in our system. We found the sensitivity obtained from the system with the unbalanced configuration was increased by 4 dB compared to the system with the balanced configuration. This is due to better utilization of optical power with our unbalanced differential detection technique.

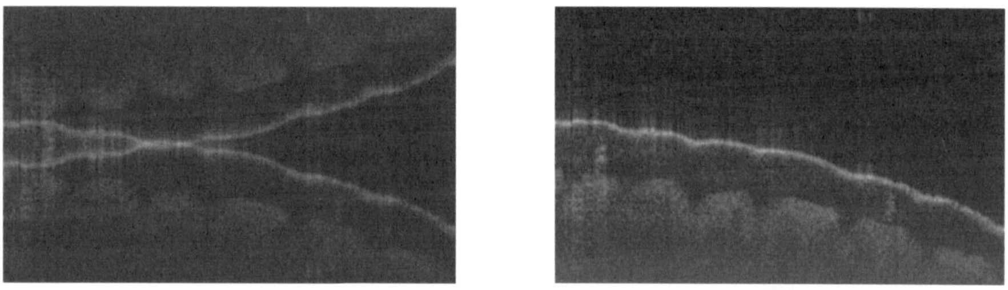

(a) (b)

Fig. 6. *In vivo* images of human finger tip acquired by our full range swept-source optical coherence tomography using the 3x3 Mach-Zehnder interferometer with unbalanced differential detection technique. (a): the image was generated using only a single detector. (b): the complex signals were used.

Fig. 6 shows *in vivo* images of a human finger tip acquired by our full range swept-source optical coherence tomography using the 3x3 Mach-Zehnder interferometer with unbalanced differential detection technique. The resolutions of the axial and lateral are 10 μm and 27 μm, respectively. The pixel size of the images is 800x900 in correspond to the image size of 3x4mm. In Fig. 6 (a), the image was generated using only a single detector, and demonstrates the folded artifact images. In Fig. 6 (b), the complex signal was used demonstrating artifact-free imaging over a depth range of 3 mm.

3. High Performance Wavelength-Swept Laser for Optical Coherence Tomography

3.1 Optical Filter Design for Swept Laser

Fig. 7 shows a schematic diagram of the FDML wavelength swept laser with a long fiber ring cavity. A SOA is used as the gain medium in the ring cavity which has a central wavelength of 1300 nm. The SOA is considered the most suitable gain medium for OCT applications: high small-signal gain, broadband gain spectra, and high relaxation resonance frequencies. The wavelength selection was achieved by a polygon-based high-speed narrowband optical scanning filter. The unidirectional wavelength sweep of a polygon scanner, as opposed to the inherently bidirectional Fabry-Perot filter, is better matched to the gain properties of an SOA. A mode-locked laser resonator was implemented using a long single mode fiber (SMF). The polygon-based reflection-type scanning narrow-bandpass filter (Yun et al., 2003) includes an optical fiber collimator, an optical diffraction grating, an afocal telescope, a polygon scanner, and a planar mirror. A collimated Gaussian beam with a broad optical spectrum from the SOA was first spread by the optical grating and then converged to the polygon by the telescope. The telescope, made of two achromatic doublets, controls both the beam size and angles. A planar mirror was placed after the polygon to reflect only the spectral component with normal incidence to the fiber. We note that the sweeping angle of the intermediate reflection from the polygon facet doubles the polygon's effective rotation angle, so that the free spectral range (FSR) of this filter is twice than when the polygon simply retro-reflects the light back to the telescope. The orientation of the grating incidence angle and the rotation direction of the polygon facet determine the direction of the wavelength tuning. The arrangement in Fig. 7 produced a unidirectional increase of the wavelength that resulted in higher optical power output. An optical fiber circulator was used to couple the light between the ring cavity and the filter. Three fiber polarization controllers were placed before the SOA, the circulator and the grating to optimize their polarization, respectively (Mao et al., 2009). The CW wavelength-swept light was coupled out of the cavity by a fiber coupler positioned after the SOA.

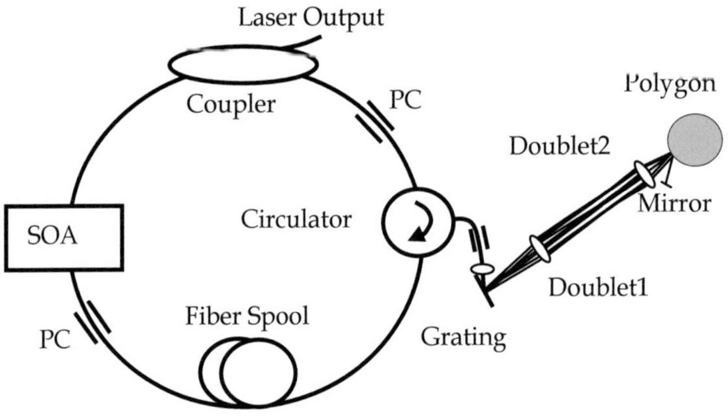

Fig. 7. Schematic diagram of a FDML wavelength-swept laser shown with a ZEMAX ray-tracing of the polygon-based narrow-band filter.

The parameters of the polygon scanning filter and its components were investigated by using a commercial optical modeling software ZEMAX (ZEMAX Development Corp., WA, USA). The ray-tracing layout of the optical filter is shown in Fig. 7 where a non-sequential ZEMAX component was used to model the polygon scanner. As the polygon was rotated clockwise by one facet, one full cycle of the continuous spectrum was swept. To achieve an optical filter with a FWHM linewidth of 0.16 nm, central wavelength of 1305 nm, free spectral range (FSR) of 110 nm, 100% duty cycle, minimum beam clipping and maximum coupling efficiency, the following optical components were chosen: a fiber collimator with 10 mm focal length and $1/e^2$ beam width of 1.89 mm, a grating with a groove frequency of 830/mm and an incident angle of 69°, two achromatic doublets with focal lengths of 75 mm and 40 mm, a polygon scanner with 72 facets and a facet area of 6.35x2.77 mm^2 (Mao et al., 2009). A summary of the input parameters and simulation results are listed in Table 1. The observed 0.5 mm chromatic focal shift after F1 on both end of the spectrum wavelength ends were compensated for our double-pass arrangement. A change of the focal spot at the image plane from circular to elliptical at the edge wavelengths, shown in Fig. 8, resulted in a nearly Gaussian output spectrum due to lower coupling efficiencies at those edges.

Input Parameter	**Value**	**Simulation Result**	**Value**
Center wavelength	1305 nm	Collimate beam width (1/e^2)	1.89 mm
Input fiber, core & NA	Single mode 9 µm & 0.11	Spectral sweeping range	± 55 nm
Collimate lens	f = 10 mm ϕ = 6mm	FWHM bandwidth at central	0.16 nm
Grating density incidence angle	830g/mm ϕ=69 deg	Diverging angle after grating at 1250 and 1360nm to central	-2.637° +2.656°
Doublet 1	$F1$ = 75 mm ϕ= 25.4mm	Converging angle at polygon at 1250 and 1360nm to central	+4.944 ° -4.979°
Doublet 2	$F2$ = 40 mm ϕ= 25.4mm	1/e^2 Beam width at Polygon	2.78 mm
Polygon facet number	72	Chromatic focal shift after F1 at 1250 and 1360nm to central	0.50 mm 0.51 mm
Polygon angle per facet	5°	Image chromatic focal shift at 1250 and 1360nm to central	< 0.1 mm < 0.1 mm
Polygon radius	31.75 mm	Image spot size at 1250, 1305, and 1360nm	120 x 10 µm^2 2.6 x 2.6 µm^2 110 x 9 µm^2
Polygon facet area	6.35x2.77mm^2	Coupling efficiency at 1250, 1305, and 1360nm	7% 38% 8%

Table 1. The parameters of the polygon scanning filter obtained from ZEMAX simulation.

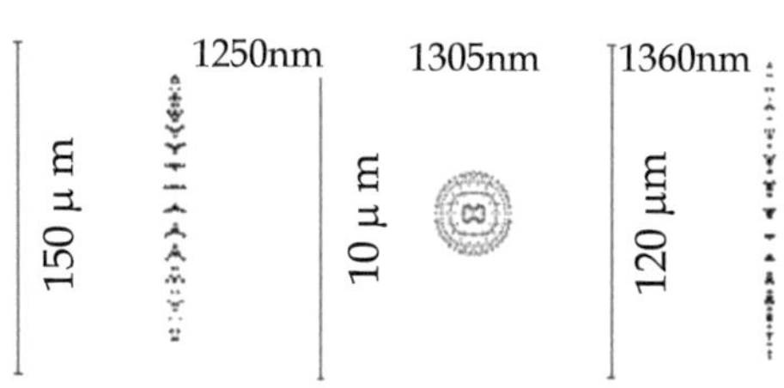

Fig. 8. Imaging spot size at 1250 nm (left), 1305 nm (central), and 1360 nm (right) of the filter from ZEMAX simulation.

The diffraction grating equation is given by (Hecht, 1979), $\lambda = (\sin\alpha + \sin\beta)/T$, where λ is the wavelength, T is the groove frequency, and α and β are the incident and the diffracted angles of the beam, respectively, with respect to the normal axis of the grating. The sweeping wavelength ($d\lambda$) could be expressed as (Yun et al., 2003):

$$d\lambda = (1/T)\cos\beta_0 (F_2/F_1)d\theta \tag{9}$$

where $d\theta$ is the sweeping angle of the polygon scanner and β_0 is the angle between the optical axis of the telescope and the grating's normal. Since $d\theta = 2\pi R dt$ for a polygon scanner, we could get a linear relationship between the sweeping wavelength and the sweeping time by integrating Eq. (9):

$$\lambda(t) = \lambda_1 + \frac{4\pi\cos\beta_0 F_2 R}{TF_1}t \tag{10}$$

Our design results in a wavelength sweeping rate of 7.31 mm/s.

3.2 Swept Laser Construction

A Fourier-domain mode-lock wavelength-swept laser based on polygon scanning filter and semiconductor optical amplifier was constructed. A high efficiency InP/InGaAsP quantum well SOA (BOA 1132, Covega) was used as the laser gain medium with a saturation output power of 19 dBm, small signal gain of 30 dB and FWHM bandwidth of 93 nm. The material structure of the quantum well active region of the SOA was optimized to increase the output power and bandwidth. A 72-facet polygon scanner (SA34, Lincoln Laser) that optimized for ultra-high speed stability was used. Two achromatic doublets (AC254-C, Thorlabs) were used to construct the telescope system. A 3.1 km optical fiber was inserted into a 5.1 m ring laser cavity as a delay line fiber to synchronize a repetition rate of 65.95 kHz of the polygon filter, which corresponds to a round-trip propagation time in the cavity of 15.16 μs. Using this setup, we could alternate between mode-locked and short cavity laser operation. In the mode-locked configuration, we used standard single mode fiber with zero dispersion around 1300 nm (SMF-130V, Prime Optical Fiber Corporation). The maximum mismatches in the roundtrip times of the different wavelengths due to dispersion and fiber birefringence were 1.1 ns and 0.4 ps, respectively. These values were calculated using a dispersion coefficient of 3.1 $ps\ km^{-1}\ nm^{-1}$ and polarization mode dispersion coefficient of 0.2 $ps\ km^{-1/2}$ of the used SMF-130V fiber. Therefore, these small time mismatches could be neglected. Three fiber polarization controllers for individually aligning polarization states of SOA, fiber circulator and grating were found to be necessary for obtaining maximum optical power. A fiber spool with 6 inch mandrel size was used in the cavity for the 3.1 km long SMF. We noticed that a fiber spool with 3 inch mandrel could reduce the optical power and flutter the laser spectrum, resulting in a reduction of the 3 dB bandwidth. This spectral fluctuation could be due to the inconsistent birefringence caused by the small bending radius of the long fiber. The ratio of the output coupler of 60/40 was used (60% of the power is coupled out), which was optimized to get the maximum optical output power.

3.3 Results and Discussions of the Swept Laser

The time-averaged normalized spectrum emitted from our FDML swept laser, measured by an optical spectrum analyzer (OSA) in peak-hold mode with a resolution of 1 nm, is shown in Fig. 9 (a). On the same graph we show a fitting of the measured spectrum to a Gaussian function, dashed line, and the spectrum obtained by ZEMAX simulations, dotted line. This simulated spectrum is the product of the filter spectrum (due to different filter coupling efficiencies at different wavelengths) and the spontaneous emission spectrum of the used SOA. A full sweeping wavelength range of 113 nm and FWHM bandwidth of 90 nm at central wavelength of 1303 nm measured from our swept laser were obtained. We note that the shape of the measured spectrum is close to a Gaussian distribution. This bandwidth of the swept laser would correspond to 8.3 μm axial resolution in the air in OCT. The measured sweeping FWHM bandwidth of the FDML swept laser was 1.43 times higher than the simulated spectrum. This increase in bandwidth is due to higher optical gains in the smaller signal range at the edge wavelengths than the central wavelength. While keeping the polygon static, two spectra were measured using the highest resolution of the OSA (0.01 nm) at the center wavelength of 1303 nm and at the dual-edge wavelengths of 1248.0 nm and 1358.2 nm, shown in Fig. 9 (b) in addition to the dynamic spectrum for comparison. A distance of 110.2 nm between the two simultaneous existing peaks corresponds to the FSR of the filter, which is in good agreement with the design specifications of FSR of 110 nm. We also note that the static spectra of our FDML swept laser had a FWHM linewidth of 0.015 nm at the central wavelength as shown in the inset of the Fig. 9 (b). The measured filter linewidth was 0.17 nm at the same wavelength as shown in the Fig. 9 (c). We found the measured laser linewidth was 11.3 times smaller than that of the filter. The linewidth of filter in the edge wavelength range increased which could be caused by the off-axis effect of the doublet; however, this effect was diminished by the FDML method as shown in Fig. (c). Fig. 9 (d) shows average output power of the swept laser versus the injection current of the SOA, which shows the laser threshold current is 100 mA.

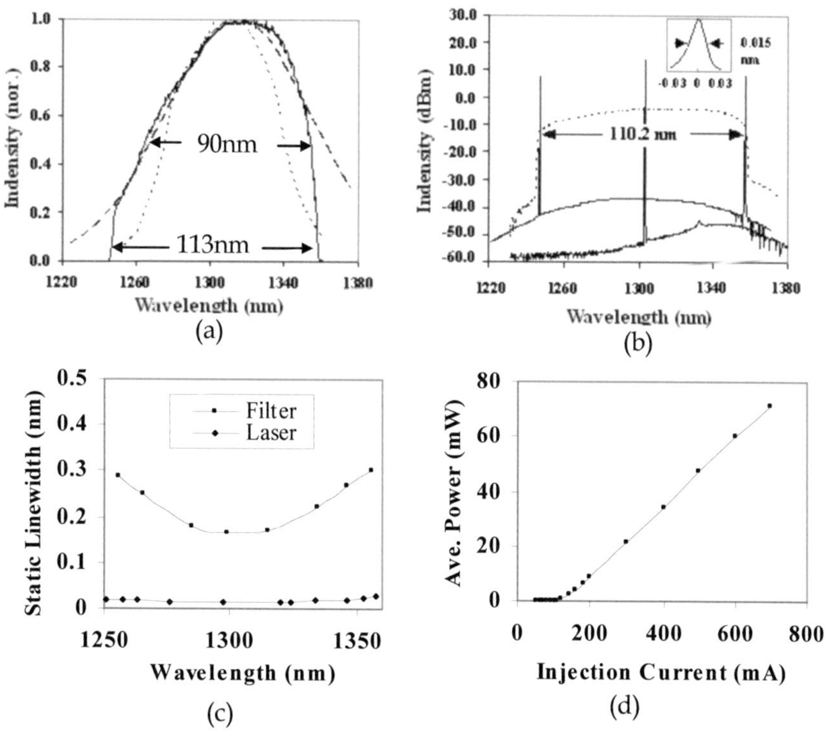

Fig. 9. (a) Measured normalized spectra of our FDML wavelength-swept laser in solid line, a

Gaussian fitting in dashed line, and simulated spectrum in dotted line. (b) Measured spectra in dBm scale with two static spectra while keeping polygon stay at the center wavelength of 1303 nm and the dual-edge wavelengths of 1248.0 nm and 1358.2 nm in solid lines. Inlet: the linear static spectrum at 1303 nm. (c) Measured static linewidth of the FDML swept-laser in comparison with measured linewidth of the polygon filter. (d) Output power versus injection current of the SOA.

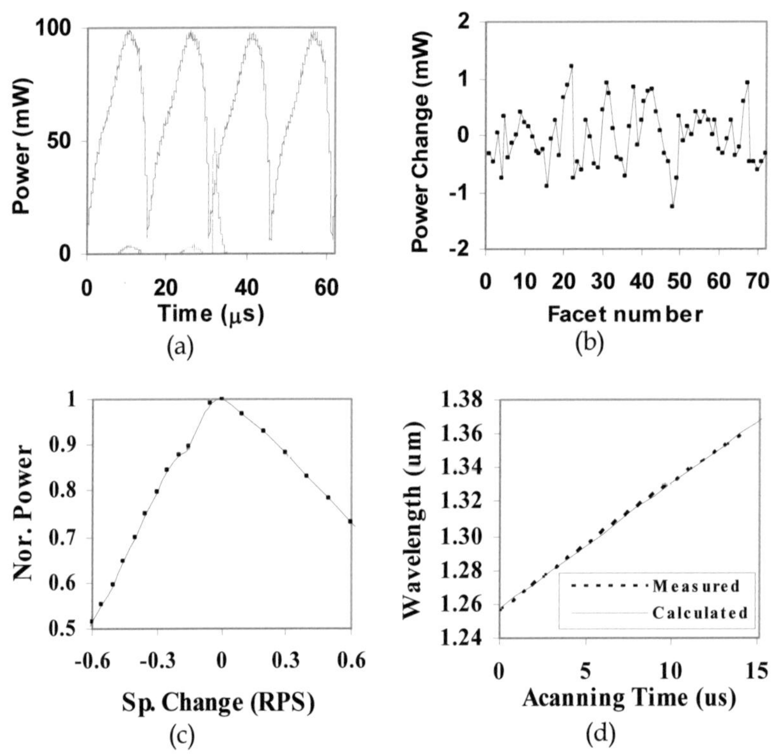

Fig. 10. (a) Oscilloscope trace of the swept laser output with four tuning cycles at a repetition rate of 65.95 kHz in solid line and a start trigger signal in dashed line. (b) Optical power change versus facet number of the polygon. (c) The normalized output power as a function of polygon speed change. (d) Theoretical and experimental wavelength swept versus time.

Fig. 10 (a) shows the measured output power of our FDML swept laser over four wavelength scans using an oscilloscope. The peak power and the average power emitted by the laser were 98 mW and 71 mW, respectively, corresponding to an SOA injection current of 700 mA. The observed scan duration of 15.16 μs with a duty cycle of 100% correspond to a repetition rate of 65.95 kHz. A wavelength start trigger signal obtained by a fiber Bragg grating (FBG) is shown in Fig. 10 (a) in dashed line, which is used for wavelength calibration and system start trigger. It will be discussed below. Laser output power change with 72 successive cycle scans were measured as shown in Fig. 10 (b). The maximum optical power change is less than 3 mW, which corresponds to a maximum 3.3% optical power fluctuation from facet to facet. Fig. 10 (c) shows the measured normalized output power of the laser as a function of the polygon rotation speed change. For this measurement, a function generator was used as an external driver to the polygon scanner. The change in the rotation speed of the polygon was obtained by adjusting the output voltage of the function generator. The laser output power was reduced when the scanner speed was either increased or decreased from the specific speed of 916 revolutions per second (RPS). More power reduction was observed when the polygon speed decreased than when it increased. This effect could be caused by the nonlinearities of semiconductor optical amplifier (Bilenca, 2006). Because the speed stability of our polygon is less than 0.02%, i.e., the speed fluctuation is less than ± 0.1 RPS, the fluctuation in the measured output power caused by the variation of the polygon speed was less than 1.0%.

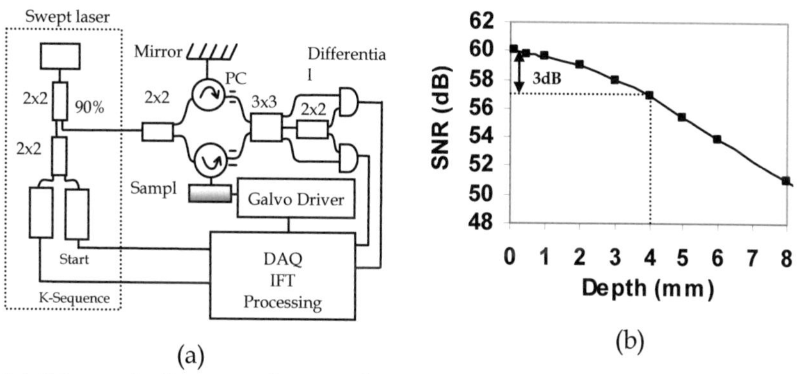

Fig. 11. (a) Schematic diagram of a complex OCT system using our swept laser with the start trigger and k-sequence. (b) The SNR of the OCT system with out swept source in the different depths.

To further characterize the properties of our swept laser for OCT application, 10% of the output power of the laser was connected to a 2x2 coupler to obtain a trigger corresponding to the start wavelength, λ_1, and a sequence of equal differences in the propagation constant k, $\Delta k = 2\pi\Delta\lambda/\lambda^2$, where $\Delta\lambda$ is the difference in wavelength. This sequence of equal valual of k is called a *k-sequence*. The start wavelength trigger for the wavelength calibration was implemented using a fiber Bragg grating with central wavelength of 1256 nm and bandwidth of 0.3 nm, a fiber circulator, and a photo-detector. The sharp rising edge of the start trigger as shown in Fig. 10 (a) in dashed line was used for the trigger of the data acquisition and wavelength calibration in the OCT system. The *k-sequence* was generated using a Mach-Zhender interferometer (MZI) with an adjustable optical path length difference and a balanced detector. By adjusting the optical path difference to about 8 mm, 1024 peaks at equal values of k were obtained. The measured wavelengths of these 1024 peaks, where Δk is equal, versus times was shown in Fig. 10 (d). We found that the measured results were in good agreement with the theoretical results calculated from Eq. 10. Using the remaining 90% of the optical output power of our swept source, we constructed a complex OCT system using a 3x3 MZI as described in the section 2 and shown in Fig. 11 (a). Measurements at different object depths were taken using a mirror and an attenuator in the sample arm. The extra background noise was subtracted by measuring the reference arm signals with the sample arm blocked. The complex interferometric signals were digitized by a data acquisition card (ATS-460, AlazarTech) with 14-bit resolution and acquired at a sampling speed of *125MS/s*. The signal data with equal-k interval were obtained by an interpolation. The start trigger signal was used to initiate the *k-sequence* and the data acquisition process for each A-scan. A-scans with resolved complex conjugate artifact were obtained by a complex inverse Fourier transformation (IFT). The signal noise ratio (SNR) versus depth was obtained by measuring point spread functions (PSF) in the different depth as shown in Fig.11 (b). PSF has a FWHM value of 8.8 μm, which agrees well with the 8.3 μm equivalent to the 3 dB bandwidth of the spectrum of the laser source. Maximum sensitivity of 114 dB was obtained by adding the attenuation in the sample arm to the SNR. To estimate the dynamic coherence length of this swept source, we observed a 3 dB drop in the amplitude of the PSF when the arm length difference was about 4 mm as shown in Fig. 11 (b). This result corresponds to an optical coherence length of 16 mm or a linewidth of 0.09 nm. We also observed a drop of 9 dB in the amplitude of the PSF at an object depth of 8 mm.

Cavity Length	3100 m (FDML)	5.1 m short cavity		
Repetition Rate (kHz)	65.95	21.5	43.8	62.1
FWHM Bandwidth (nm)	90	84.6	79.0	71.4
Coherence Length (mm)	16	14	12	10
Average Power (mW)	71	62	50	42

Table 2. Comparison of the performance of our FDML laser with 5.1m short cavity laser

To get a better understanding of the operation of our FDML swept laser, we switched the laser to the shorter cavity. Table 2 shows a comparison of the FWHM spectral bandwidth, instantaneous coherence length and average output power of our FDML swept laser operating at 65.95 kHz repetition rate to that of the short cavity swept laser operating at 21.5 kHz, 43.8 kHz, and 62.1 kHz repetition rates, respectively. In this short cavity laser, when the repetition rate increases, the laser performance is deteriorated, for example, when the repetition rate increases from 21.5 kHz to 62.1 kHz, the FWHM spectral bandwidth, instantaneous coherence length and average output power decreases from 84.6 to 71.4 nm, 14 to 10 mm, and 62 mW to 42 mW, respectively. In comparison, the FWHM bandwidth, coherence length, and average output power of our FDML swept laser reaches 90 nm, 16 mm, and 71 mW at 65.95 kHz repetition rate, respectively. From these results, the FDML technique in the swept laser source has proved to be an effective method for enhancing the overall performance of the swept laser.

4. Fiber Probes for Optical Coherence Tomography Imaging

4.1 Design of fiber probes

Fiber-based OCT system has capability of using an optic fiber probe. The light beam usually is guided through a SMF and is focused on a tested sample by an optical lens attached to the SMF. Back-reflected light carrying information about the sample is coupled back into the fiber, and then signal detection and data processing systems will collect the useful information for imaging. The optic probe is one of the crucial parts of OCT imaging system. The beam profile, i.e. working distance (focal distance from lens surface), depth of field (two times the Raleigh range), and spot size (waist diameter) of the optical probe in the sample will directly determine the properties of the image such as image location, depth, and resolution. Thus, image quality and light coupling efficiency from the sample will be directly influenced by the beam quality of the probe. For the best optical performance of a probing lens, its beam profile must be designed to be consistent with the light penetration depth in the sample. In most biomedical imaging systems, light from the probe will be directed into a turbid tissue. Based on interaction properties of light with turbid tissue (Sainter et al., 2002) the range of penetration depth is from 0.5-3 mm at near infrared wavelengths. For example, the penetration depths are 0.7 mm and 3.0 mm in human skin and liver respectively at 1300 nm, a conventional wavelength used in OCT systems. Thus, for designing an optical probe, working distance should be in the range of 0.4 – 1.2 mm in the air that depends on the tissues to be tested. There is a tradeoff between the depth of field and beam spot size because the depth of field of a lens is positively related to the square of the spot size according to the theory of Gaussian beam. A large depth of field unavoidable results in a large spot size. Thus, the optimal depth of field is in the range of 0.8 - 1.5 mm in the air; this keeps the spot size in the range of 26 - 35 μm at the 1300 nm wavelength. For an ultra-small optical lens, it is not possible to achieve a large working distance by directly attaching a lens to a SMF because of the strong focus ability of lens and the small mode field diameter (MFD) of the SMF. A fiber spacer with a homogeneous index of refraction has to be added between the SMF and the lens for beam expansion prior to focusing to obtain a larger working distance. Therefore, theoretical modeling becomes necessary to obtain a fiber lens with optimized optical beam performance for imaging different tissues.

In this section, we study two types of fiber lenses, GRIN and ball fiber lenses. We used ZEMAX to design both GRIN and ball fiber lenses by choosing an appropriate surface type and analysis method.

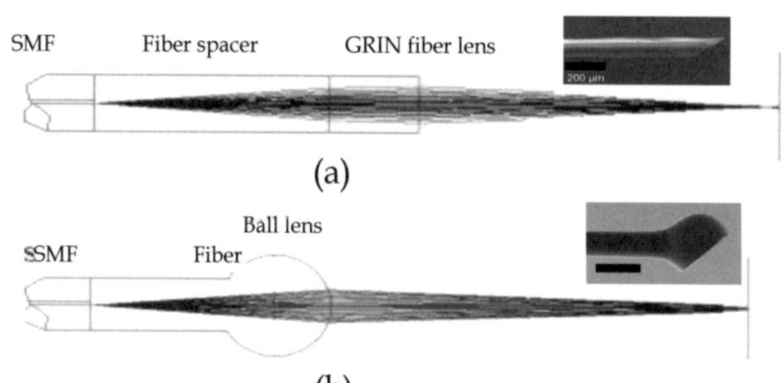

Fig. 12. ZEMAX layouts of ray trace for the GRIN (a) and ball (b) fiber lens systems, respectively. Insets: scanning electron micrographs of the GRIN and ball fiber lens tips fused with angle-polished beam director, respectively. Marks are 200 μm.

For a GRIN fiber lens, the gradient surface type used in ZEMAX will depend on the profile of the refractive index. The refractive index profile of the GRIN fiber lens used in this work is a radial index gradient, which is very similar to that of a conventional glass GRIN (or called SELFOC) lens. The index of refraction is highest in the center of the lens and decreases with radial distance from the axis. The following quadratic equation closely describes the refractive index of a GRIN fiber lens (Kogelnik & Li, 1966; Emkey & Jack, 1987):

$$n(r) = n_0(1 - \frac{g^2}{2} r^2) \quad (11)$$

where r is the radial position from the axis, n_0 is refractive index on the lens axis, g is the gradient constant. The pitch, $p = 2\pi/g$, is the spatial period of the ray trajectory. For modeling of the ball fiber, the Standard Surface type in ZEMAX is employed. Fig. 12 (a) and (b) show the ZEMAX ray trace layout of the GRIN and ball fiber lenses, respectively, with their scanning electron micrographs in the insets. The working distance, depth of field and spot size were calculated in ZEMAX using the Gaussian beam theory. The theoretical results will be shown and discussed in comparison with the experimental results below.

4.2 Fabrication Method of the fiber probes

The GRIN and ball fiber lens probes were made from a standard Corning SMF-28 single mode fiber as the principal light guide, a fiber spacer and a GRIN or a ball fiber lens as the focusing lens. For the GRIN lens probe, a fiber spacer with same outer diameter (0.125 mm) as SMF-28 was fusion-spliced via arc welds to the Corning SMF-28 and then accurately cleaved to a theoretically-determined length. A GRIN fiber was then fusion-spliced to the cleaved fiber spacer and precisely cleaved at a pre-calculated length to generate a desired beam-distance profile (i.e., working distance, depth of field, and spot size). For a short working distance probe, the section of the fiber spacer was omitted resulting in a simple fabrication process. For the ball lens probe, a fiber spacer was fusion-spliced via arc welds to the Corning SMF-28 and then accurately cleaved to a theoretically-determined length plus extra 0.2 mm. The tip of the fiber spacer then was fused via arc welds to a perfect ball shape by inputting an appropriate fusion setting. To ensure minimum back-reflection for both probes, the indexes of the fiber spacer and the center of GRIN fiber were matched to the core index of the SMF.

We used a conventional low cost off-the-shelf optical multi-mode GRIN fibers as the GRIN lens, which has 0.1 mm core size, 0.14 mm outer diameter, a core refractive index $n_0 = 1.487$, and a gradient constant $g = 3.76$ at 1300 nm (Prime Optical Fiber Corp., Taiwan). The fiber spacers (Prime Optical Fiber Corp., Taiwan) are made of pure silica without a core. Fusion-splicing was processed using an Ericsson FSU 995 fusion-splicer and an EFC11 fiber cleaver (3SAE Technologies, TN, USA). The spliced interfaces produced minimum back-reflections since the mechanical strength at the interface was similar to that of the untreated fiber. The desired focused beam profile was obtained by tailoring the length of the fiber spacer and parameters of fiber lenses (length of GRIN fiber and diameter of the ball) based on the theoretical results. We fabricated the different variations of the GRIN and ball fiber lens modules with the different length of the fiber spacer and the different lens parameter. All samples were listed in Table 3 with detailed information.

A beam profile measurement system (BeamView Analyzer, OR, USA) with an infrared camera (Electrophysics, NJ, USA) and a Super Luminous Diode source (Covega, MD, USA) with 60nm 3dB bandwidth at 1310 nm center wavelength was used to characterize the beam parameters of the lens system. A 40X JIS microscopic objective lens and a related objective tube were attached to the input window of the camera to increase the image resolution. The horizontal and vertical resolutions of the system were 1.0 μm and 1.1 μm, respectively. The distribution of light intensity at various distances along the direction of propagation after the lens was accurately measured by the beam profile system. Working distance, depth of focus, $1/e^2$ spot size, and Gaussian fitting were analyzed from the measured intensity distribution. The results demonstrated in this work are all in the air medium.

In addition, after characterization of the lens, a beam director could be attached to the lens for a side-view probe. The different attaching methods were used for the two lenses. For the GRIN lens, a fiber spacer was fusion-spliced to the finished lens end as a beam director by polishing the end of the fiber spacer to a 45 degrees angle and coating the polished surface with a total reflection film. This then allowed the beam to be reflected at a 90 degrees angle creating a side-view probe. For the ball lens probe, the beam can be 90-110 degree reflected by a 45-50 degree polished face on the ball lens by the total internal reflection. Insets of Fig. 12 (a) and (b) show the typical scan electron microscope (SEM) pictures of the GRIN and ball fiber lens tip fused with beam directors, respectively. The fiber lens tip together with a tubing system and a connected linearly scanning or 360 degrees rotated motor could be built as an endoscope, or catheter, or a needle probes. The diameter of these probes could be as small as 0.4 mm which is best suitable for internal *in situ* and *in vivo* biomedical imaging, diagnostic, guided surgery, and treatment with a minimal invasion.

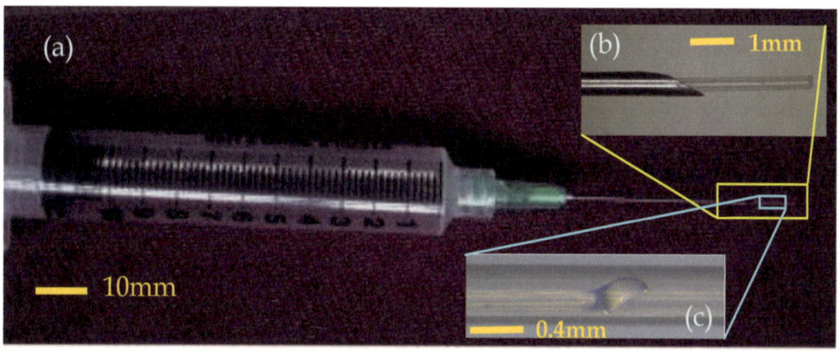

Fig. 13. OCT side-view needle probe showing the tubing and angle-polished ball lens. (a) needle probe. (b) retracted needle tip with protective tubing. (c) protective tubing and exposing the lens.

As a sample, a needle probe designed for the OCT imaging in this work is shown in Fig 13 (a). The lens and the uncoated portion of the SMF are protected in a transparent inner catheter (OD 0.49 mm) shown in Fig. 13 (b, c). The buffered portion of the fiber is attached to an outer flexible catheter after the syringe (OD 1.4 mm), which is fastened onto a modified syringe piston, while the transparent inner catheter is inserted into a 21 G (OD 0.81 mm) echogenic spinal needle (VWR, Mississauga, ON, Canada). After insertion into the tissue, the needle can be drawn back while the optical probe stays inside of the tissue as shown in Fig. 13 (b). The probe is then scanned axially inside the tissue driven by a linear scanner, such that a two dimensional OCT image is formed. If a fiber GRIN lens is used, the size of the inner catheter could be as small as 0.4 mm because the diameter of the GRIN lens is smaller than the fiber ball lens.

Sp.#	Length of Fiber Spacer (mm)	Fiber Lens		Measured Beam Properties		
		Type/Diameter (μm)	Length (mm)	Working Distance (mm)	Depth of Field (mm)	Spot Size (μm)
1	0	GRIN100/140	0.60	0.18	0.16	13
2	0	GRIN100/140	0.55	0.20	0.30	16
3	0	GRIN100/140	0.52	0.28	0.50	22
4	0	GRIN100/140	0.50	0.38	0.60	23
5	0	GRIN100/140	0.48	0.41	0.85	25
6	0	GRIN100/140	0.46	0.40	1.30	30
7	0	GRIN100/140	0.45	0.38	1.45	32
8	0.48	GRIN100/140	0.17	1.00	0.95	28
9	0.48	GRIN100/140	0.16	1.10	1.5	35
10	0.48	GRIN100/140	0.145	1.20	1.8	41
11	0.48	GRIN100/140	0.14	1.05	2.0	45
12	0.52	Ball Lens/300	~	1.00	3.6	50
13	0.55	Ball Lens/300	~	1.4	2.1	45
14	0.62	Ball Lens/300	~	1.20	1.1	27
15	0.70	Ball Lens/300	~	1.00	0.5	20
16	0.74	Ball Lens/300	~	0.90	0.33	16

Table 3. Structures of the various fiber lenses with measured beam properties.

4.3 Characterization Results of the fiber probes

The measured results of the beam properties are listed in Table 3 along with detailed descriptions of the listed samples. For each sample, optical intensity distribution data on the radial (i.e. x and y) planes were collected along the beam propagation (i.e. optical axial z) direction from the plane of the first half peak intensity (begin-plane), through the maximum intensity plane, i.e. focus plane (center-plane), to the second half peak intensity plane (end-plane). Beam properties including working distance, spot size, and depth of field were analyzed by measured intensity distribution data with distance from the lens surface to the focal plane, $1/e^2$ beam diameter at the focal plane, and the distance between the begin-plane and the end-plane, respectively. The theoretical and experimental results of working distance, depth of focus, and spot size of different variations vs. length of GRIN fiber or diameter of the ball lens (bottom x-axis), and length of fiber spacer (top x-axis) are shown in Fig. 14 (a), (b), and (c), respectively, where, lines represent the theoretical results from ZEMAX at 1300 nm, amount them, dark doted line represent GRIN fiber lens without a fiber spacer, dark and light solid lines represent GRIN fiber lens with a constant length of fiber spacer (0.48 mm) and a constant length of GRIN fiber (0.17 mm), respectively; dark and light dash lines represent ball fiber lens with a constant length of fiber spacer (0.62 mm) and a constant diameter of the ball (0.30 mm), respectively. The experimental results were represented by points, amount them, triangle points represent GRIN fiber lens and square points represent the ball lens.

From the theoretical result shown in Fig. 14, short working distance (<0.4 mm) could be obtained by the GRIN fiber lens without fiber spacer shown as the dark dotted lines. To obtain larger working distance, a fiber spacer has to be used. In these cases, the working distance varies sharply with the length of GRIN fiber for the GRIN fiber lens and with the diameter of the ball for the ball fiber lens, but it varies less sharply with the length of the fiber spacer. The working distances have saturated values for each case. By compensating the working distance with the depth of field and the spot size, the optimized parameters (i.e. 0.9 - 1.2 mm working distance, 0.9 – 1.1 mm depth of filed, and <30 μm spot size) are not at the position of the largest working distance, instead, the optimized positions are around 0.17 mm length of the GRIN fiber with 0.48 mm length of fiber spacer for GRIN fiber lens and 0.3 mm diameter of ball and 0.62 mm length of fiber spacer for ball fiber lens. The results of the experimental results as shown in Fig. 14 and Table 3 indicated that the ZEMAX numerical optical design software were in a good agreement with the experimental results. We obtained the working distance of 1.0 mm, the depth of field of 0.95 mm, and the spot size of 28 μm from a GRIN fiber lens module (sample #8) and the working distance of 1.2 mm, the depth of field of 1.1 mm, and the spot size of 27 μm from a ball fiber lens module (sample #14).

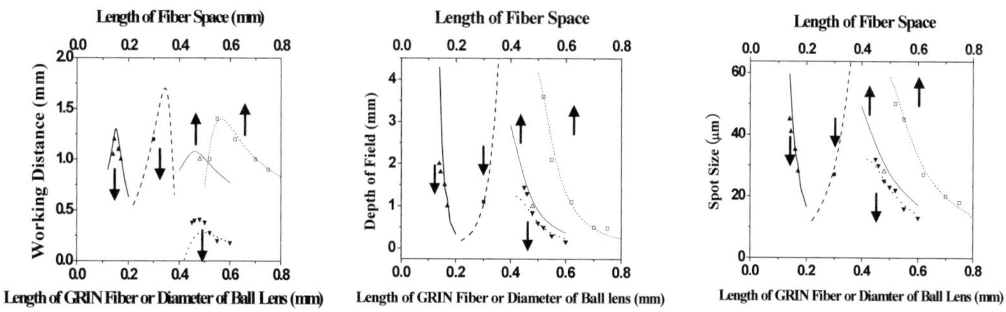

(a) (b) (c)

Fig. 14. Theoretical and experimental results of working distance (a), depth of field (b), and spot size (c) vs. length of GRIN fiber or diameter of the ball lens (bottom x axis), and length of fiber spacer (top x axis), where, lines represent the theoretical results from ZEMAX at 1300 nm, amount them, dark doted line represent GRIN fiber lens without a fiber spacer, dark and light solid lines represent GRIN fiber lens with a constant length of fiber spacer (0.48 mm) and a constant length of GRIN fiber (0.17 mm), respectively; dark and light dash lines represent ball fiber lens with a constant length of fiber spacer (0.62 mm) and a constant diameter of the ball (0.30 mm), respectively. The related experimental results were represented by the points.

We found quality of the beam depends very much on the quality of the surface cleaving and the alignment of the fusion-splicing between the fiber spacer and the fiber lens. The high quality beam is easier to obtain for the probe with the ball fiber lens because the ball is made from the fiber spacer and there is no interface between the fiber spacer and the ball lens. By well controlling the cleaving and the fusion-splicing, we obtained high quality of beam for the probe of the GRIN fiber lens as well. Fig. 15 shows measured and Gaussian-fitted $1/e^2$ intensity beam diameters along the axial distance z (zero is the position of the lens surface) at x (horizontal) and y (vertical) radial coordination in the distance range of depth of field for the samples #1, #3 and #8 with the GRIN fiber lenses as shown in Table 3.

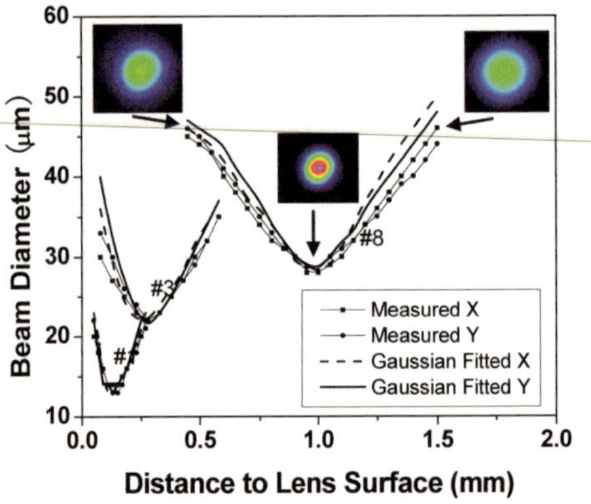

Fig. 15. Measured and Gaussian-fitted $1/e^2$ intensity beam diameters along the axial distance (zero is the position of the lens surface) at x (horizontal) and y (vertical) radial coordination in the distance range of depth of field of the samples #1, #3 and #8, which was made from the GRIN fiber lens. Insets: the cross-section beam profiles at three planes for the sample #8.

For each curve in Fig. 15, the smallest beam diameter value presents the spot size, x-coordinate value at the pole point indicates the working distance, and the distance range of the curve indicates the depth of field. The working distance of 0.18 mm, depth of field of 0.16 mm, and spot size of 13 μm were obtained for the sample #1 with 0.60 mm length of 100/140 GRIN fiber lens which was directly attached to SMF without fiber spacer. If the length of GRIN fiber was reduced to 0.52 mm, the beam became less converged resulting the three parameters increased slightly to 0.28 mm, 0.5 mm, and 22 μm, respectively. When a 0.48 mm fiber spacer was inserted between SMF and GRIN fiber and the length of GRIN fiber is reduced to 0.17 mm, significant less converged beam is observed. The working distance of 1.0 mm, depth of field of 0.95 mm, and spot size of 28 μm were obtained for sample #8.

The measured beam diameters are well matched to Gaussian-fitted values in the center (focused) regions, but have small deviations in the two edge side regions as shown in Fig. 15. The insets in Fig. 15 shown images of the cross-section beam profile at begin, center, and end planes, respectively, for the sample #8. The circular shapes of the profile images indicate high x and y symmetry of the beam profiles through all the range of depth of filed.

Considering chromatic aberrations, from ZEMAX simulation for the ball fiber lens in the wavelength range of 1260 - 1370 nm, the relative variations of the working distance, depth of field and spot size were calculated all smaller than 4.0%. For the GRIN fiber lens, the range of the zero-dispersion wavelengths, $\{\lambda_0\}$ is 1297-1316 nm. The zero-dispersion slope, S_0, equal to or smaller than 0.101 ps/nm^2-km. Using the standard formula of fiber dispersion, $D(\lambda) = S_0[\lambda - \lambda_0^4 / \lambda^3]/4$ (ps/nm-km), we calculated the changes of refractive index in the 1260 - 1370 nm wavelength range. By using these values in ZEMAX, we calculated the relative changes of the working distance, depth of field and spot size were all smaller than 3%. Based on our results, the desired beam profile for the application of optical biomedical imaging systems can be obtained by the GRIN and ball fiber lens with or without fiber spacers. The technique described here possesses a high degree of flexibility for designing ultra-small optical probes with different beam shapes for the different tissue imaging.

5. OCT Imaging

Fig. 16 (a) and (d) show SS-OCT images of human finger *in vivo* taken using fiber probes # 14 (working distance, depth of field and spot diameter of 1.2 mm 1.1 mm, and 27 μm) and # 16 (working distance, depth of field and spot diameter of 0.9 mm 0.33 mm, and 16 μm) acquired by our catheter-based complex SS-OCT using our 3x3 Mach-Zehnder interferometer with unbalanced differential detection technique with image size of 5x2mm. The image depth shown in Fig. 16 (a) is slightly larger than that in Fig. 16 (b), but the image is blurrier in Fig. 16 (a) than that in Fig. 16 (b), which taken by the probe with larger depth of field and spot size. The image shown in Fig. 16 (b) has higher resolution than that in Fig. 16 (a), which can be seen clearly with finer structures in layer of epidermis (grey arrow), sweat gland (white arrow), and blood vessel in subcutis layer (black arrow).

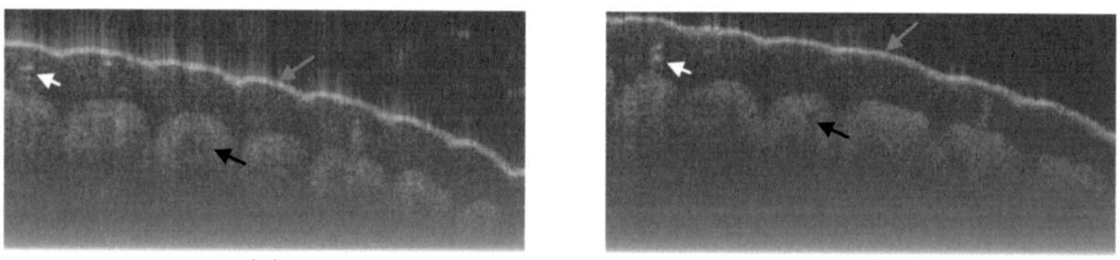

(a) (b)

Fig. 16. *In vivo* human finger SS-OCT images taken with probe #14 (working distance, depth of field and spot diameter of 1.2 mm 1.1 mm, and 27 μm) and # 16 (working distance, depth of field and spot diameter of 0.9 mm 0.33 mm, and 16 μm) acquired by our catheter-based complex SS-OCT using our 3x3 Mach-Zehnder interferometer with unbalanced differential detection technique with image size of 5x2mm.

Fig. 17 shows *ex vivo* images of coronary artery of rabbit with forward-view (a, b) probe with ball lens #16 and side-view (c, d) probe with GRIN lens #5 acquired by our catheter-based complex SS-OCT using our 3x3 Mach-Zehnder interferometer with unbalanced differential detection technique with image size of 2.5x2mm by scanning the probe along the artery (a, c) and scanning cross the artery (b, d). Three layers of tunica intima, tunica media, and tunica adventitia for the coronary artery are viewed clearly as indicated by the gray, black, and white arrows in all four images in Fig. 17. The fine layers of muscle and elastic fiber in the tunica media of the coronary artery are shown obviously in the images obtained by scanning the probe cross the artery.

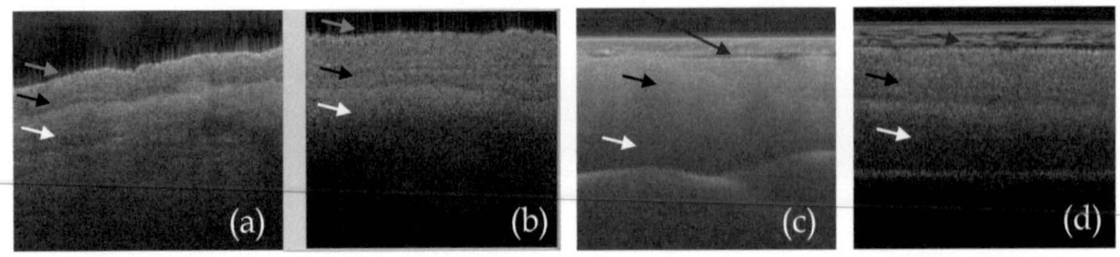

Fig. 17. *Ex vivo* images of coronary artery of rabbit scanning along the artery (a, c) and scanning cross the artery (b, d) with forward-view probe (a, b) with ball lens #16 and side-view (c, d) probe with GRIN lens #5 acquired by our catheter-based complex SS-OCT using our 3x3 Mach-Zehnder interferometer with unbalanced differential detection technique.

Fig. 18 shows *ex vivo* images of heart atrium (a, b), artery (c) of mice, and heart atrium (d, e, f) of pig with forward-view probe with ball lens #16 acquired by our catheter-based complex SS-OCT using our 3x3 Mach-Zehnder interferometer with unbalanced differential detection technique with image size of 2x2mm. The shapes and structures of these internal organs of small and large animals are viewed clearly from these OCT images.

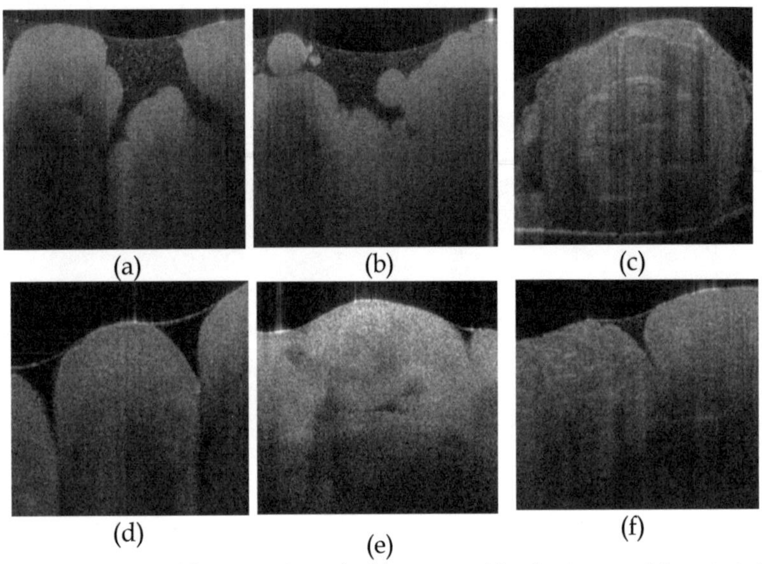

Fig. 18. *Ex vivo* images of heart atrium (a, b), artery (c) of mice, and heart atrium (d, e, f) of pig acquired by our catheter-based complex SS-OCT using our 3x3 Mach-Zehnder interferometer with unbalanced differential detection technique.

The *in vivo* and *ex vivo* OCT images shown in Fig. 16, 17, and 18 indicate that our catheter-based complex SS-OCT system is capable of imaging the biomedical tissues or the inside organs for human, small and big animals and it is most suitable for applications of diagnosis and guided surgery.

6. Acknowledgments

Authors gratefully thank Dan P. Popescu and Michael G. Sowa from Institute for Biodiagnostics of National Research Council of Canada, and Tim Cheung from Heart Institute of University of Ottawa for their providing of the animal tissues.

7. Conclusion

We have demonstrated a catheter-based full range swept-source optical coherence tomography system. A 3x3 quadrature Mach-Zehnder interferometer with a new unbalanced differential detection method for SS-OCT have been firstly presented. Using this setup, a complex conjugate artifact suppression of 27 dB has been achieved. A 90° phase shift between the two interferometric outputs was obtained thereby eliminating the need for further trigonometric calculations. Also, our setup resulted in a 4 dB increase in the signal-to-noise ratio compared to a similar interferometer with the commonly used balanced detection technique. We have then demonstrated a high-performance wavelength-swept laser that uses a high-efficiency semiconductor optical amplifier, a high-speed polygon-based narrowband scanning filter, and a Fourier domain mode lock technique. This laser produced 71 mW average output power with an instantaneous linewidth of 0.09 nm, and it could be tuned over a wavelength range of 113 nm at a repetition rate of 65.95 kHz. We also constructed an OCT system that uses our laser source where we have shown that its parameters are optimized for this application. We presented next the design, construction and beam profile characterization of different variations of graded-index and ball fiber lenses, which were recently proposed for ultra-small probes for OCT imaging. Those fiber lens modules were made of single mode fibers and GRIN and ball fiber lenses with/without fiber spacers between them. We used fusion-splicing in between the fibers, lenses and spacers to ensure high quality light transmission. We found that beam-distance profiles (i.e. 0.4 - 1.2 mm of focus distance, 0.8 – 1.5 mm of depth of field, and 26 – 35 μm of spot size) can be obtained by precisely adjusting the lengths of the fiber spacer and the GRIN fiber lens or diameter of the ball lens for the different tissue imaging in human beings and animals. We obtained very high quality focused Gaussian beam profiles with high x and y symmetry using the conventional multi-mode GRIN fibers and home-made fiber ball lenses. Their high quality beam and ultra-small size make such fiber lens based probes very valuable for biomedical optical imaging systems. The *in vivo* and *ex vivo* OCT images acquired by our catheter-based full range SS-OCT system indicate that this system is capable of imaging the biomedical tissues or inside organs for human, small/big animals and it is most suitable for applications of diagnosis and guided surgery.

8. References

Bilenca, A. et al. (2006). Numerical study of wavelength-swept semiconductor ring lasers: the role of refractive-index nonlinearities in semiconductor optical amplifier and implications for biomedical imaging application, *Opt. Lett.* 31, 760-762, ISSN: 0146-9592.

Chinn, S.R.; Swanson, E. A. & Fujimoto, J. E. (1997). Optical coherence tomography using a frequency-tunable optical source, *Opt. Lett.*, 22, 340-342, ISSN: 0146-9592.

[a]Choma, M.A. et al. (2003). Sensitivity advantage of swept source and Fourier domain optical coherence tomography, *Opt. Exp.* 11, 2183-2189, ISSN: 1094-4087.

[b]Choma, M.A.; Yang, C. & Izatt, J.A. (2003). Instantaneous quadrature low-coherence interferometry with 3x3 fiber-optic couplers, *Opt. Lett.* 28, 9672162-2164, ISSN: 0146-9592.

De Boer, J.F. et al. (2003). Improved signal-to-noise ratio in spectral-domain comared with time-domain optical coherence tomography, *Opt. Lett.* 28, 2067-2069, ISSN: 0146-9592.

Diaz-Sandoval, L. J. (2005). Optical Coherence Tomography as a tool for percutaneous coronary interventions, *Catheter. And Cardio. Interventions,* 65, 492-496, ISSN: 1522-1946.

Emkey W. L. & Jack, C. A. Analysis and evaluation of graded-index fiber-lenses, *J. of Lightwave Tech.*, LT-5, 1156-1164, ISSN:0733-8724.

Fercher, F. et al. (1995). Measurement of intraocular distances by backscattering spectral interferometry, *Opt. Commun.* 117, 443-448, ISSN: 0030-4018.

Fujimoto, J. G. et al. (1999) High resolution in vivo intra-arterial imaging with optical coherence tomography, *Heart,* 82, 128-133,.

Hausler, G. & Lindner, M. W. (1998). Coherence Radar and Spectral Radar - new tools for dermatological diagnosis, *J. Biomed. Opt.* 3, 21-31, ISSN: 1083-3668.

Hecht, E. (1997) *Opics* (Addison-Wesley, Reading, Mass.).

Huang, D. et al. (1991). Optical coherence tomography, *Science,* 254, 1178-1181, ISSN: 0036-8075.

Huber, R. et al. (2005). Amplified, frequency swept lasers for frequency domain reflectometry and OCT imaging: design and scaling principles, *Opt. Exp.*, 13, 3513-3528, ISSN: 1094-4087.

Huber, R.; Adler, D.C. & Fujimoto, J.G. (2006). Buffered Fourier domain mode locking:unidirectional swept laser sources for optical coherence tomography imaging at 370,000 lines/s, *Opt. Lett.* 31, 2975-2977, ISSN: 0146-9592.

Huber, R.; Wojtkowski, M. & Fujimoto, J.G. (2006) Fourier domain mode locking (FDML): a new laser operating regime and applications for optical coherence tomography, *Opt. Exp.* 14, 3225-3237, ISSN: 1094-4087.

Jafri, M. S. et al. (2005) Optical coherence tomography in the diagnosis and treatment of neurological disorders, *J. Biomed. Opt.* 10(5) 051603, ISSN: 1083-3668.

Kogelnik, H. W. & Li, T. (1966) Laser Beam and Resonators, *Appl. Opt.* 5, 1550, ISSN: 0003-6935.

Leitgeb, R.; Hitzenberger, C.K. & Fercher, A.F. (2003). Performance of Fourier domain vs. time domain optical coherence tomography, *Opt. Exp.* 11, 889-894, ISSN: 1094-4087.

Li, H. et al. (2006). Feasibility of interstitial doppler optical coherence tomography for in vivo detection of microvascular changes during photodynamic therapy, *Lasers in Surgery and Medicine* 38, 754–761, ISSN:0196-8092.

Li, X. et al. (2000). Imaging needle for optical coherence tomography, *Opt. Lett.* 25, 1520-1522, ISSN: 0146-9592.

Mao, Y. et al. (2007) Graded-index fiber lens proposed for ultrasmall probes used in biomedical imaging, *App. Opt.*, 46, 5887-5894, ISSN: 0003-6935.

[a]Mao, Y. et al. (2008). 3x3 Mach-Zehnder Interferometer with Unbalanced Differential Detection for Full Range Swept-Source Optical Coherence Tomography, *Appl. Opt.* 47, ISSN:2004-2010.

[b]Mao, Y. et al. (2008) Design and Implementation of Fiber Lenses for Ultra-Small Probes Used in Biomedical Imaging, *Proc. SPIE*, 6826, 68261A, ISSN: 0277-786X.

Mao, Y. et al. (2009). High Performance Wavelength-Swept Laser with Mode-Locking Technique for Optical Coherence Tomography, *Opt. Comm.*, 282, 88-92, ISSN:0030-4018.

Oh, W. Y. et al. (2005). 115 kHz tuning repetition rate ultrahigh-speed wavelength-swept semiconductor laser, *Opt. Lett.* 30, 3159-3161, ISSN: 0146-9592.

Oh, W. Y. (2008). Speed polarization sensitive optical frequency domain imaging with frequency muliplexing, *Opt. Exp.* 16, 1096-1103, ISSN: 1094-4087.

Podoleanu, A. Gh. (2000). Unbalanced versus balanced operation in an optical coherence tomography system, *Appl. Opt.* 39, 173-182, ISSN:2004-2010.

Priest, R. G. (1982) Analysis of fiber interferometer utilizing 3x3 fiber coupler, *IEEE Trans. Microwave Theory Tech*, MTT-30, 1589-1591, ISSN:0018-9480.

Rao, B. et al. (2007). Investigation of coherence amplification with a semiconductor optical amplifier employed in a swept source OCT system, *Proc. of SPIE*, 6429, 642924-1, ISSN: 0277-786X.

Reed, W. A.; Yan, M. F. & Schnitzer, M. J. (2002). Gradient-index fiber-optic microprobes for minimally invasive *in vivo* low-coherence interferometry, *Opt. Lett.* 27, 1794-1796, ISSN: 0146-9592.

Rollins, A. M. & Izatt, J. A. (1999). Optimal interferometer designs for optical coherence tomography, *Opt. Let.*, 24, 1484-1486, ISSN: 0146-9592.

Sainter, A. W.; King, T. A. & Dickinson,V Theoretical comparison of light sources for use in optical coherence tomography, *Proc. SPIE* 4619, 289-299, ISSN: 0277-786X.

Sarunic, M.V. et al. (2005). Instantaneous complex conjugate resolved spectral domain and swept-source OCT using 3x3 fiber couplers, *Opt. Exp.* 13, 957-967, ISSN:1094-4087.

Sarunic, M.V.; Applegate, B.E. & Izatt, J.A. (2006). Real-time quadrature projection complex conjugate resolved Fourier domain optical coherence tomography, *Opt. Lett.* 31, 2426-2428, ISSN: 0146-9592.

Sheem, S. K. (1981) Optical fiber interferometers with [3x3] directional couplers: analysis, *J. Appl. Phys.* 52, 3865-3872, ISSN:0021-8979.

Shishkov, M.; Bouma, B. E. & Tearney, G. J. (2006). System and method for optical coherence tomography, *U.S. Patent* 20060067620A1 (Mar. 30).

Sticker, M. et al. (2001). Quantitative differential phase measurement and imaging in transparent and turbid media by optical coherence tomography, *Opt. Lett.* 26, 114-116, ISSN: 0146-9592.

Swanson, E. (2002). Ultra-small optical probes, imaging optics, and methods for using same, *U.S. Patent* 6445939 (Sept. 3).

Takada, K. et al. (1987). New measurement system for fault location in optical waveguide devices based on an interferometric technique, *App. Opt.* 26, 1603-1606, ISSN: 0003-6935.

Tran, P. H. et al. (2004). *In vivo* endoscopic optical coherence tomography by use of a rotational microelectromechanical system probe, *Opt. Lett.* 29, 1236-1238, ISSN: 0146-9592.

Vakoc, B.J.et al. (2006) Elimination of depth degeneracy in optical frequency_domain imaging through polarization-based optical demodulation, *Opt. Lett.* 31, 362-364, ISSN: 0146-9592.

White, B. R. et al. (2003). In vivo dynamic human retinal blood flow imaging using ultra-high-speed spectral domain optical coherence tomography, *Opt. Exp.* 11, 3490-3497, ISSN: 1094-4087.

Yang, V. X. D. et al. (2005). Endoscopic Doppler optical coherence tomography in human gastrointestinal tract: initial experience, *Gastrointest. Endosc.* 61, 879-890, ISSN: 0016-5085.

Yang, V. X. D. et al. (2005). Interstitial Doppler optical coherence tomography, *Opt. Lett.* 30, 1791-1793, ISSN: 0146-9592.

Yazdanfar, S.; Rollins, A. M. & Izatt, J. A. (2000) Imaging and velocimetry of the human retinal circulation with color Doppler optical coherence tomography, *Opt. Lett.* 25, 1448-1450, ISSN: 0146-9592.

Youngquist, R. C.; Carr, S. & Davies, D. E. N. (1987). Optical coherence-domain reflectometry: A new optical evaluation technique, *Opt. Lett.*, 12, 158-160, ISSN: 0146-9592.

[a]Yun, S.H. et al. (2003). High-speed optical frequency-domain imaging, *Opt. Exp.* 11, 2953-2963, ISSN: 1094-4087.

[b]Yun, S. H. et al. (2003). High-speed wavelength-swept semiconductor laser with a polygon-scaner-based wavelength filter, *Opt. Lett.* 28, 1981-1983, ISSN: 0146-9592.

Yun, S.H. et al. (2004). Removing the depth-degeneracy in optical frequency domain imaging with frequency shifting, *Opt. Exp.* 12, 4822-4828, ISSN: 1094-4087.

Zhang, J. et al. (2004). Full range polarization-sensitive fourier domain optical coherence tomography, *Opt. Exp.* 12, 6033-6039, ISSN: 1094-4087.

[a]Zhao, Y. et al. (2000). Phase-resolved optical coherence tomography and optical Doppler tomography for imaging blood flow in human skin with fast scanning speed and high velocity sensitivity, *Opt. Lett.* 25, 114-116, ISSN: 0146-9592.

[b]Zhao, Y. et al. (2000). Doppler standard deviation imaging for clinical monitoring of *in vivo* human skin blood flow, *Opt. Lett.* 25, 1358-1360, ISSN: 0146-9592.

3

Brain Imaging and Machine Learning for Brain-Computer Interface

Maha Khachab, Chafic Mokbel, Salim Kaakour,
Nicolas Saliba and Gérard Chollet*
University of Balamand
Lebanon
**Ecole Nationale Supérieure des Télécommunications*
Paris

1. Introduction

Human-computer interfaces are in continuous development, from keyboard, mouse, touch screen, to voice dictation, gesture recognition, etc. The aim is to facilitate the interaction between the human brain and the resources offered by a machine or a computer. Recently, a wider interest has emerged in directly interfacing the brain and the computer. The development of methods that combine the nervous system with artificial devices is attracting a growing interest from clinical research, because the interaction between brain and machines may lead to novel prosthetic devices or to a more efficient use of computer resources by breaking the barriers imposed at present by the classical human-machine interfaces. Individuals with impaired motor control may be disabled in the performance of their daily activities. Their motor performance, however, can be supported by artificial motor control systems. Such motor support systems may also assist healthy individuals in performing their tasks. One can also imagine interacting with different systems in parallel, or developing newer software tools without the need to physically typing the code.

The brain output pathway allows it to interact through its natural biological interfaces. In order to design a system to support an impaired human motor control function or to directly interact the brain with computers and machines, one should address the method of interfacing with the human body. The interface should provide signals from the human body to derive motor intention. These interfaces and technologies are studied in the wide domain of neurotechnology. Neurotechnology is a multidisciplinary domain that integrates, not exclusively, knowledge and scientific evidence from neurosciences, engineering, and signal processing. The present chapter focuses specifically on Brain-Computer Interfaces.

P. Sajda et al., defines (Sajda et al., 2008) the Brain-Computer Interface (BCI) as: "A Brain-Computer Interface is a system that includes a means for measuring neural signals from the brain, a method/algorithm for decoding these signals and a methodology for mapping this decoding to a behavior or action". The system is thus formed of three principal blocks. The first two blocks are critical for the success of the BCI. Actually, the neural signals to be measured have to be chosen adequately and the decoding of these signals should be accurate. The use of the output of the decoder in the third block of a BCI application is a pure engineering problem. This block should take into account some specific aspects related to the errors that a BCI system may lead to and the particular context of a BCI. This chapter focuses on the first two blocks, i.e. the acquisition and decoding of neural signals.

Informative neural signals may be collected at the microscopic level (e.g. spike trains), mesoscopic level (e.g. electrocorticogram) and/or, macroscopic level (e.g. electroencephalogram). In order to collect the spike trains, electrodes are generally implanted in a surgery with non negligible risk. BCI approaches based on these signals are invasive approaches. Besides the high surgical risks, such approaches have to face other challenges. The power consumption is a key issue limiting the possibility of advanced processing in the electrode implantation area. Therefore, neural signals have to be transmitted out of the implantation area which by itself is also a challenge.

Clearly, non-invasive approaches, e.g. EEG signals-based systems, are more attractive than the invasive ones for the limited risk they may incur. However, signals in non invasive approaches are less precise than the spike trains measured in electrode-based approaches. Advanced processing is therefore required in the decoding block.

In this chapter, we focus mainly on the non-invasive approaches for BCI. Several techniques have been proposed to measure relevant features from EEG or MRI signals and to decode the brain targets from those features. Such techniques are reviewed in the chapter with a focus on a specific approach. The basic idea is to make the comparison between a BCI system and the use of brain imaging in medical applications. Actually, based on neural signals like EEG, the electro-magnetic activity at the surface of the cortex may be measured. A practitioner would make use of such images of the cortex surface to detect abnormalities or diseases. The chapter shows this parallelism and how it has been exploited to build a state of the art BCI system.

After a brief description of a general BCI system, a brief review of the neural signals and their measurements is provided. A particular focus is on EEG signals. EEG is a standard non-invasive and nearly risk-free method that has been extensively used in medical applications. In order to decode the signals collected, feature extraction is first performed. Based on the relevant features computed, a classification is performed. State of the art feature extraction approaches systems are presented in the chapter. Brain imaging techniques allow to visualize the surface of the cortex. This suggests using brain imaging techniques to evaluate the electro-magnetic activity at the cortex surface that will define a vector of features. These features will be given to the decoding/classification algorithm as input. At the output of the classification algorithm, the decoded intention would be detected. The chapter presents briefly several techniques for brain imaging with a focus on subspace correlation methods. These methods are detailed in the chapter.

Several classifiers, e.g. Artificial Neural Networks (ANN), Independent Component Analysis (ICA) and other approaches have been used extensively in BCI systems. As an example both the Support Vector Machine (SVM) and the Gaussian Mixture Model (GMM) are presented.

To illustrate the concepts presented, a BCI system is described and some experimental results are provided. The system makes use of signal subspace decomposition as feature extraction and support vector machine as classifier. The chapter provides some hints about the system implementation before providing conclusions and perspectives.

2. BCI System

The basic design and operation of a BCI system include the following components (Veltink et al., 2001)(Wolpaw et al., 2002)(Ebrahimi et al., 2003):

1. **Signal acquisition and digitization**: The input is the EEG activity or brain signals from the user. This input is acquired by recording electrodes, amplified, and digitized. As stated above the signal acquisition defers largely from invasive and noninvasive approaches.

2. **Signal processing**: It comprises two stages:
   a. Feature extraction: Features related to specific electrophysiology components are extracted.
   b. Decoding algorithm: It translates the signal features into device commands that accomplish the user's request.

3. **Output device**: In general, the output device may be prosthesis with its control system or a video screen. The output is the feedback the brain uses to maintain and improve communication or to control prosthesis.

4. **Operating format**: It guides the operation (onset, offset, and timing) of the BCI.

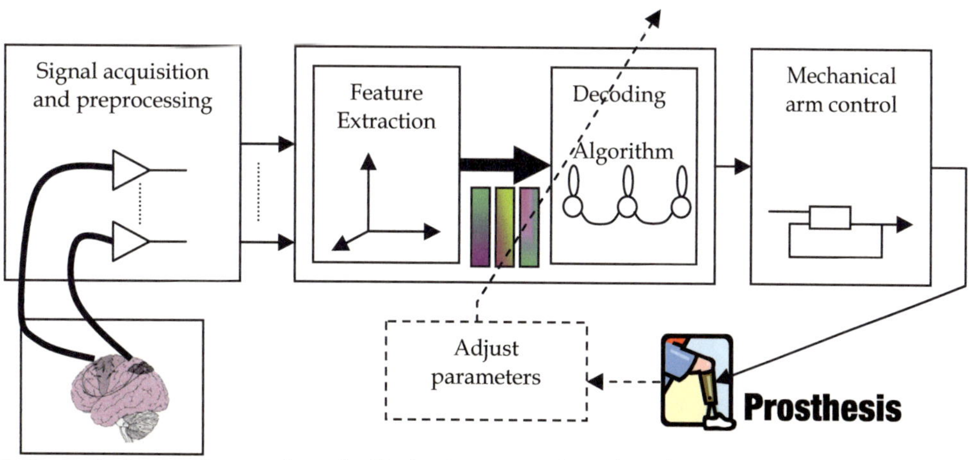

Fig. 1. Basic design and operation of a Brain-Computer Interface (BCI).

3. Feature Extraction

Several measurement procedures have been used in modern BCI. As stated earlier, they can be divided into two categories. Non invasive procedures include Electroencephalography (EEG), Magnetoencephalography (MEG), functional magnetic resonance imaging (fMRI), positron emission tomography (PET) and near infrared spectroscopy (NIRS). Electrocorticography (ECoG), a method in which signals are recorded using intracranial electrodes, is used as an invasive procedure to collect signals.

3.1 Spike Signals

The brain has a fascinating design consisting of a huge number of neurons that operate in parallel and a distributed memory system formed of synapses. There are over 100 trillions of synapses in the cerebral cortex. Each neuron is assumed to produce a unique and consistent spike waveform which is difficult to detect. The duration of a spike is on average 1 millisecond and its peak-to-peak voltage is from 100 to 400 μV. The spikes cannot be used directly by the detection part of a BCI system. State of the art invasive BCI systems, start by sorting the spike trains (Shenoy et al., 2006). The distribution of specific spike signals can be used in order to detect the desired movement or intention.

3.2 Non-Invasive Signals

Non-invasive exploration of human brain functions has always been a central topic in biomedical research. This is not only motivated by the high risk of invasive implantation surgery but also because macroscopic information has inherent value due to the information it provides on the motor command. Before any movement occurs, motor commands carried by descending motor pathways must first be organized in the brain. The target of the movement is identified by pooling sensory information in the posterior parietal cerebral cortex (Jakson et al., 1999). This information is then transmitted to the supplementary motor and premotor areas where a motor plan is developed. The plan includes information about the specific muscles that need to be contracted, the strength of contraction, and sequence of contraction. The motor plan is implemented by commands transmitted from the primary motor cortex through the descending pathways. Successful execution of these motor commands, however, depends on feedback provided to the motor cortex through the ascending pathways to the somatosensory cortex as well as through the visual pathway. One should also add that during both the planning and execution stages of a movement, motor processing is also provided by 2 major control systems, the cerebellum and basal ganglia (Figures 2 and 3).

In order to monitor the spatio-temporal evolution of the cortical activity within the human brain, several methods make use of the electric potential and/or magnetic fields associated with the intracellular current that flows within the active pyramidal cells of the cortex. Surface electrodes can record electrical potential differences from a scalp surface leading to what is called electroencephalography (EEG). Magnetoencephalography (MEG) makes use of a superconducting quantum interference device (SQUID) magnetometer in order to record the weak magnetic fields outside the head surface (Knuutila *et al* 1993). Moreover, one goal in electric and magnetic recordings is to form an image of the electrical sources distributed across the cortex (Mosher et al., 1992) (Dale & Sereno, 1993).

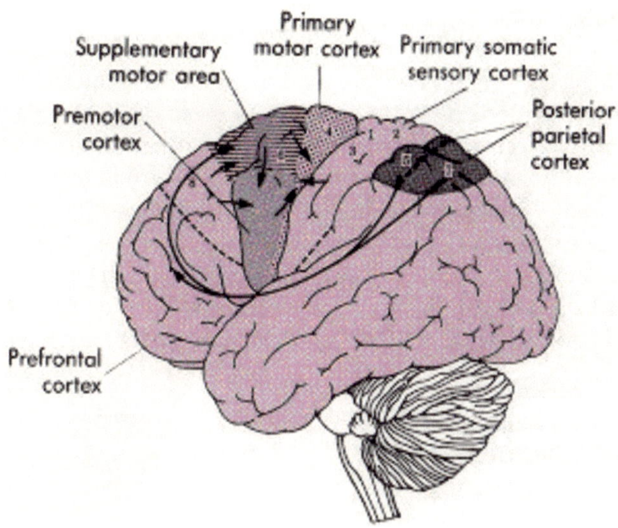

Fig. 2. Cortical projections involving the motor areas. (From (Berne RM, Levy MN, Koeppen BM, Stanton BA. *Physiology*, Fourth edition, 1998).

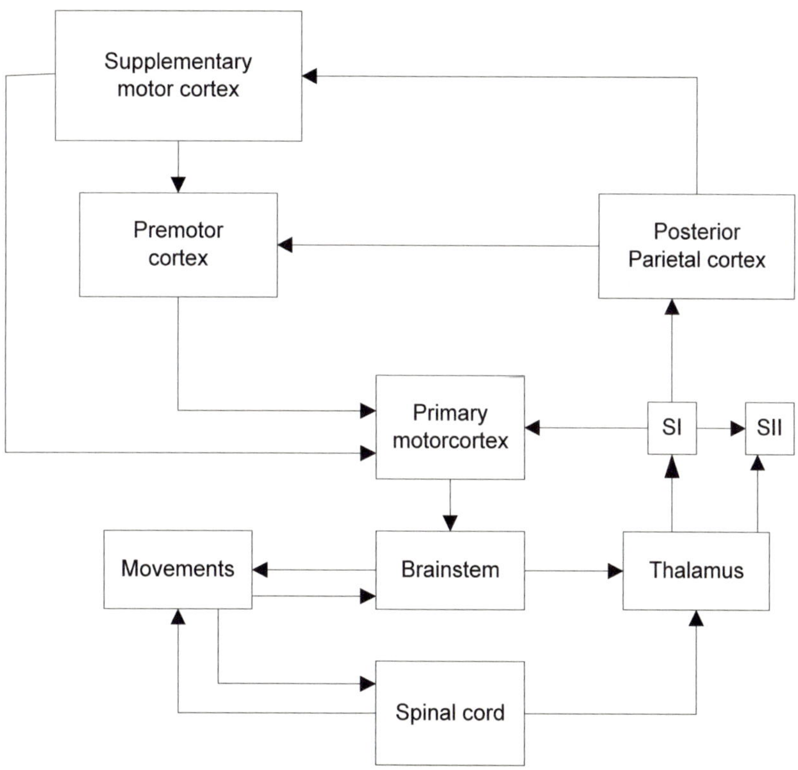

Fig. 3. Flow diagram showing the sequence of activity in the voluntary motor and somatosensory feedback pathways. (From Berne RM, Levy MN, Koeppen BM, Stanton BA. *Physiology*, Fourth edition, 1998).

3.2.1 Electroencephalography

The EEG is a recording of the rhythmic electrical activity that can be made from the cerebral cortex via electrodes placed on the surface of the skull. In clinical neurology, EEG is recorded from a grid of standard recording sites. EEG is recorded as a potential difference between a signal or active electrode (electrode that records the activity at the site of interest on the surface of the skull) and a reference or indifferent electrode (e.g. electrode placed at the ear lobe) (Westbrook, 2000). A conductive paste will be used to decrease contact impedance and electrode migration (Westbrook, 2000).

Different EEG standard exist and mainly differ in the position of the electrodes on the skull. In the international 10-20 system EEG signals are recorded from a 59 electrodes placed on the skull as shown in Fig. 4 (Sajda et al., 2003). The signals are usually referenced to the left mastoid.

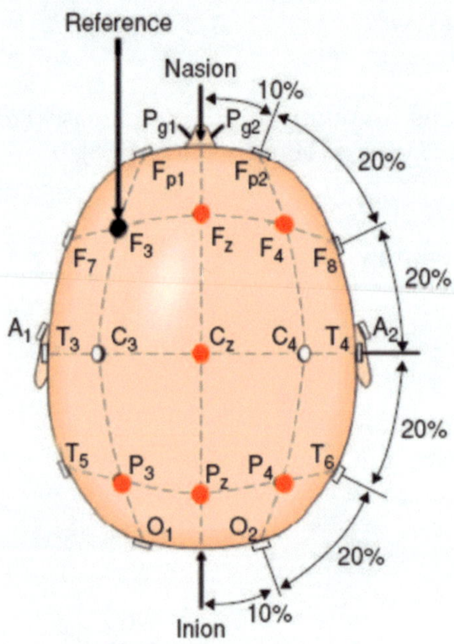

Fig. 4. The International 10-20 electrodes placement system (From Jasper HH. The ten-twenty electrode system of the international federation. In: Internal Federation of Societies for Electroencephalography and Clinical Neurophysiology. Recommendations for the practice of clinical electroencephalography. Elsevier, 1983: 3-10).

EEG patterns are characterized by the frequency and amplitude of the electrical activity (Westbrook, 2000). The normal human EEG shows activity over the range of 1-30 Hz with amplitudes in the range of 20-100 μV. The observed frequencies have been divided into several groups:

- Alpha (8-13Hz): Alpha waves of moderate amplitude are typical of relaxed wakefulness and are most prominent over the parietal and occipital sites.
- Beta (13-30 Hz): Lower amplitude beta activity is more prominent in frontal areas and over other regions during intense mental activity. They are associated with an

alert state of mind and can reach frequencies near 50 hertz during intense mental activity.

- Delta (0.5-4 Hz): Delta waves are normal during drowsiness and early slow-wave sleep
- Theta (4-7 Hz): Theta waves arise from emotional stress, especially frustration or disappointment.
- Mu (8-12 Hz): Mu waves are linked to cortical motor activity and have been associated with beta activity. Mu waves diminish with movement or the intention to move. They occupy the same frequency band as Alpha waves.
- Gamma (26-40 Hz): Gamma waves are considered to reflect the mechanism of consciousness.

These waves, especially Mu and Beta, have been used as features in several BCI systems. An example of EEG waves is provided in Fig. 5.

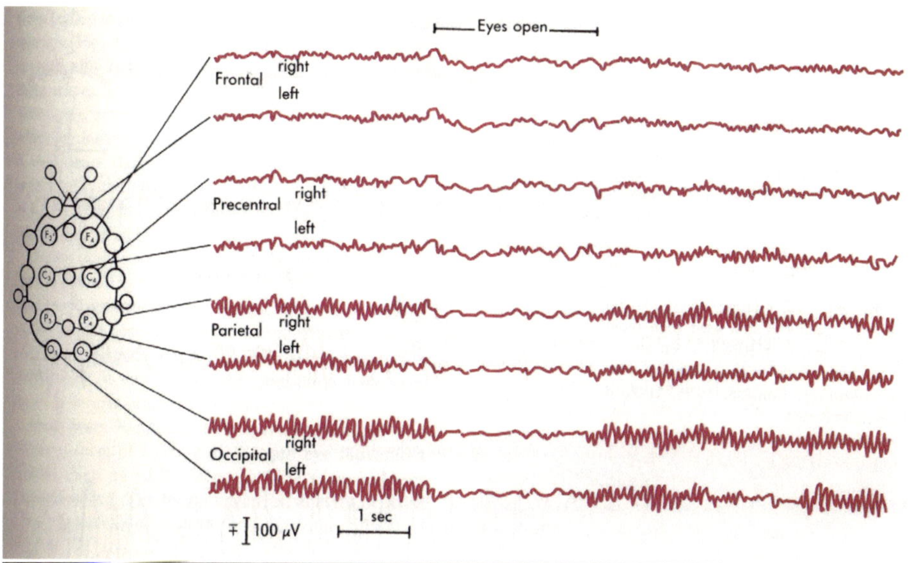

Fig. 5. EEG in a normal resting awake human. The recordings were made from eight channels at the same time. The electrode positions are indicated. (From Berne RM, Levy MN, Koeppen BM, Stanton BA. *Physiology,* Fourth edition, 1998).

The importance of the EEG resides in its ability to describe the activity on the cortex surface. Therefore, several techniques of brain imaging proposed the use of EEG in order to provide a full image of the electrical activity on the surface of the cortex. Based on the EEG signals, different sets of features can be derived. Classical features used in different BCI systems are first briefly described. Brain Imaging based features are then provided in detail.

3.2.2 EEG-Based Classical Features

Several features have been classically derived from the EEG data and used by the decoding algorithm (Hammon & de Sa, 2007). The key idea is to derive some relevant and robust features from the EEG signals that would reliably represent the task to be detected. Time and frequency analysis of the EEG signals are used to derive such features.

EEG patterns frequency based features
The patterns described above, i.e. delta, theta, alpha/mu, beta and gamma (26-40Hz), may be used as features. Classical filters or Fast Fourier Transform permit to compute those patterns and their corresponding energies in the analysis window. Those energies define the feature vector that is used at the input of the decoding process. Advanced techniques make use of filter banks in order to determine the energies of the above patterns.

Wavelet transform features
Wavelet transform permits to apply an adequate filter bank on signals. Compared to classical filter banks, wavelet transform offer a more precise analysis since the time window is selected depending on the analysis frequency band leading to a more precise analysis. Several types of wavelets, Symlet, Daubechies and Coiflet, (Darvishi & Al Ani, 2007) (Xu et al. 2007) (Hammon et al., 2008) have been successfully used in state of the art BCI systems.

Autoregressive models features
Autoregressive (AR) modeling has been used successfully in several domains. A p-order AR model consists in predicting the current sample of the signal from a linear combination of the previous p samples. This leads to an all-pole model in the z-transform domain and the corresponding parametric spectrum can be determined. Estimating the linear combination coefficient in the model is generally done in order to minimize the prediction error following the minimum mean square error criterion. Several efficient algorithms are available to solve this estimation problem (Kay 1999).
In BCI, both simple autoregressive (Hammon & de Sa, 2007) and multivariate autoregressive (Anderson et al., 1998) models have been experimented with satisfactory results.

Independent Component Analysis features
Principal component analysis (PCA) has been used with success to extract independent components from multi-electrode EEG signals (Lagerlund et al., 1997). Independent component analysis (ICA) has been proposed as an improvement of the PCA (Hyvarinen & Oja, 2000) (Vorobyov & Cichoki, 2002). Kohonen LVQs have been also used for this purpose (Pregenzer & Pfurtscheller, 1999).

3.2.3 EEG-Based Brain Imaging Features

As stated earlier EEG is particularly useful in BCI, because EEG has a short time constant and is a relatively simple, inexpensive, and noninvasive procedure. Although EEG frequency bands give a general description of brain activity, EEG signals provide additional information to estimate electrical activity at the cortical surface. Several approaches have been proposed and successfully experimented to visualize the electrical activity at the cortex surface. This is part of the brain imaging field. Brain imaging is often used by practitioners in order to detect diseases.
As discussed previously, the electrical activity on the cortex surface also reflects the movement to be executed. Therefore, it has been proposed (Khachab et al., 2007) to use brain imaging techniques in order to extract reliable features for the decoding process of a BCI

system. The underlying idea is to consider a grid representing the cortical surface and compute the electrical activity in every point of this grid. This provides relevant features for the BCI system.

Several approaches for source imaging exist (Jung et al., 2001) (Gavit et al., 2001) (Rajapakse & Piyaratna, 2001) (Michel et al., 2004). While they may be all experimented in the case of BCI, the MUSIC-like brain imaging techniques (Mosher & Leahy, 1998, 1999) have been selected for their robustness. This approach is briefly represented here.

Consider a current dipole located at a position $\vec{r}$ on the cortical surface and with a moment vector $\vec{q}$. This dipole creates (Sajda et al., 2003) a voltage potential v at the sensor position $\vec{s}$ such as:

$$v = \vec{g}(\vec{s}, \vec{r}).\vec{q} \tag{1}$$

where $\vec{g}(.)$ is the lead vector.

Assume p the current dipole sources. The voltage for n time instances is recorded simultaneously at m sensors. The spatio-temporal data matrix can be written as:

$$\begin{pmatrix} v_1(t_1) & \cdots & v_1(t_n) \\ \cdots & \cdots & \cdots \\ v_m(t_1) & \cdots & v_m(t_n) \end{pmatrix} = \begin{pmatrix} \underline{g}^T(\underline{s}_1, \underline{r}_1) & \cdots & \underline{g}^T(\underline{s}_1, \underline{r}_p) \\ \cdots & \cdots & \cdots \\ \underline{g}^T(\underline{s}_m, \underline{r}_1) & \cdots & \underline{g}^T(\underline{s}_m, \underline{r}_p) \end{pmatrix} . \begin{pmatrix} \underline{q}_1(t_1) & \cdots & \underline{q}_1(t_n) \\ \cdots & \cdots & \cdots \\ \underline{q}_p(t_1) & \cdots & \underline{q}_p(t_n) \end{pmatrix} \tag{2a}$$

or equivalently,

$$\underline{\underline{V}} = \left[\underline{\underline{G}}(\underline{r}_1) \cdots \underline{\underline{G}}(\underline{r}_p)\right] \underline{\underline{Q}}^T = \underline{\underline{G}}.\underline{\underline{Q}}^T \tag{2b}$$

where $\underline{\underline{G}}(\underline{ri})$ represents the matrix of raw lead vectors associating the ith source dipole and the m sensors, and where $\underline{\underline{Q}}$ is the matrix whose j^{th} column represents the time series of the moment of the jth dipole source.

Brain imaging or localization of current sources on the cortical surface can be seen as the solution to Eq. 2 where the current sources positions and moments are unknown (Mosher & Leahy, 1999). This is obviously a nonlinear problem with no direct solution. The complexity is increased by the fact that the measured voltage at the sensors includes some measurement noise. Including measurement noise, Eq. 2 becomes:

$$\underline{\underline{V}} = \underline{\underline{G}}.\underline{\underline{Q}}^T + \underline{\underline{E}} \tag{3}$$

where $\underline{\underline{E}}$ designates the measurement noise matrix.

The measurement noise is supposed to be zero-mean and white and not correlated with the useful signals, i.e. the $\underline{\underline{R}}_{ee} = \sigma_e^2.\underline{\underline{I}}$ is a diagonal autocorrelation matrix. Moreover, the orientations of the moments of the current sources are assumed to be time-invariant. Let us consider the autocorrelation function of the voltage measurement, it can be estimated using:

$$\underline{\underline{R}}_V \cong \frac{1}{n} \underline{\underline{V}}.\underline{\underline{V}}^T = \frac{1}{n} \underline{\underline{G}}.\underline{\underline{Q}}^T.\underline{\underline{Q}}.\underline{\underline{G}}^T + \sigma_e^2.\underline{\underline{I}} \tag{4}$$

Applying singular value decomposition leads to:

$$\underline{\underline{R}}_V = \Phi_S \Lambda_S + n\sigma_e^2 \underline{\underline{I}} \tag{5}$$

where Φ_S corresponds to the first *p* eigenvectors.

A least square estimation of the current sources consists in minimizing the cost function:

$$\min\|E\|^2 = \min\left\|\underline{\underline{V}} - \underline{\underline{G}}\,\underline{\underline{Q}}^T\right\|^2 = \min\left\|\underline{\underline{V}} - \underline{\underline{G}}\,\underline{\underline{G}}'\,\underline{\underline{Q}}^T\right\|^2 \quad (6)$$

where $\underline{\underline{G}}'$ is the pseudo inverse of the gain matrix $\underline{\underline{G}}$.

Eq 6 is clearly non linear and would require high computational search in order to find a solution. The "MUltiple SIgnal Classification" (MUSIC) has been proposed in (Schmidt 1981) to reduce the complexity of this search. The MUSIC algorithm is briefly introduced hereafter in terms of subspace correlations. Given the rank of the Gain matrix *p* and the rank of the signal matrix F_s that is at least equal to *p*, the smallest subspace correlation value represents the minimum subspace correlation between principal vectors in the Gain matrix and the signal subspace matrix F_s. The subspace of any individual column g_i with the signal subspace will exceed this smallest subspace correlation. While searching the parameters, if the minimum subspace correlation approaches unity, then all the subspace correlations approach unity. Thus, a search strategy of the parameter set consists in finding *p* peaks of the metric:

$$subcorr^2 = \frac{\underline{g}^T \hat{\Phi}_S \hat{\Phi}_S^T \underline{g}}{\|\underline{g}\|} \quad (7)$$

The gain vectors $\underline{g}$ are considered for all points of a grid that represents the cortical surface. The point of the grid with the highest subcorrelation coefficient is selected and the algorithm may tries to have a fine detection of the dipole around this point or restart looking for the next dipole. However, and for the BCI system, the algorithm is stopped at the first stage and a feature vector is built including all the subspace correlations obtained in the different points of the grid. This vector is then used as input for the decoding process of the BCI system.

The computation of the subspace correlation coefficients is performed on the points of a grid representing the cortical surface of the brain. Two grids have been studied: the first, a spherical grid defined to be 1 cm inside the skull; the second, a grid with no analytical form designed to follow, at 1cm distance, the skull. For the nonanalytic grid, the skull has been divided into layers on the z-axis. In every layer, the grid is defined as an ellipse that is 1cm distant from the skull position. For a few layers, skull points were lacking to precisely define the ellipse. In such cases points were borrowed from adjacent layers and a linear interpolation is performed to estimate the required skull point.

The present study uses the MUSIC-like brain imaging techniques of signal subspace correlations and metrics to localize brain activity positions (Mosher & Leahy, 1999). Two pattern recognition algorithms have been tested as classifiers: the artificial neural network multilayer perceptron and the support vector machines. Experiments have been conducted on subject 1 of a reference database (NIPS 2001 Brain Computer Interface Workshop) (Sajda et al., 2003) .

4. Classifiers or Decoding Process

Several classifiers have been used in BCI systems. Two principal classifiers are presented here: Artificial neural network (ANN) and Support Vector Machines (SVM).

4.1 Artificial Neural Network (ANN)

ANN, specifically the MultiLayer Perceptron (MLP), has been successfully used as a classifier in BCI systems. The units of computation in an ANN is called neuron, in reference to the human neuron it tries to simulate. These neurons are elementary machines that apply a nonlinear function, generally a sigmoid or a hyperbolic tangent, to a biased linear combination of its inputs. If $x_1, \ldots, x_l$ are the neuron input and y is its output, we can write:

$$y = f\left(\sum_{k=1}^{l} a_k x_k + b\right) \qquad (8)$$

where $f(\,)$ is the neuron function, b is the bias and $\{a_k\}$ are the linear combination weights representing the synapses connections.

In the MLP structure, neurons are organized in layers. The neural units in a layer do not interact with each other. They take their inputs from the neurons of the preceding layer and provide their output to the neurons of the next layer. In other words, the outputs of neurons of layer i-1 excite the neurons of layer i. Therefore, MLP is completely defined by its structure and the connections weights. Once defined, the ANN parameters, the weights for each neuron, must be estimated. This is usually done according to a train set and using the gradient descent algorithm. In the train set, it is supposed available the inputs and desired outputs of the MLP for different experiments. The gradient descent will iteratively adjust the MLP parameters so as to have its output the closer to the desired output for the different experiments.

4.2 Support Vector Machines (SVM)

SVM is a recent class of classification and/or regression techniques based on the statistical learning theory developed in (Vapnik, 1998). Starting from simple ideas on linear separable classes, the case of linear non-separable classes is studied. The separation of classes using linear separation functions is extended to the nonlinear case. By projecting the classification problem to a higher dimension space, high performance non-linear classification may be achieved. In the higher dimension space, linear separation functions are used while the passage to this space is done with a non-linear function. Kernel functions permit to implement this solution without needing the mapping function or the dimension of the higher space. More detail is provided in (Cristianini & Taylor, 2000). In (Khachab et al., 2007) several kernel functions have been used and compared.

5. Experiments

5.1 Database

Experiments have been conducted on subject 1 of a reference database from the NIPS 2001 Brain Computer Interface Workshop (Sajda et al., 2003). The "EEG Synchronized Imagined Movement" database was considered. The task of the subjects was to synchronize an indicated response with a highly predictable timed cue. Subjects were trained until their responses were within 100 ms of the synchronization signal. Eight classes of trials (explicit or imagined for left/right/both/neither) were randomly performed within a 7 minute 12 seconds block. Each block is formed of 72 trials. A trial succession of events is shown in Fig. 6. The EEG was recorded from 59 electrodes placed on a site corresponding to the International 10-20 system and referenced to the left mastoid. In a preprocessing stage, artifacts were filtered out from the EEG signals (Ebrahimi et al., 2003), and signals were sampled at 100 Hz.

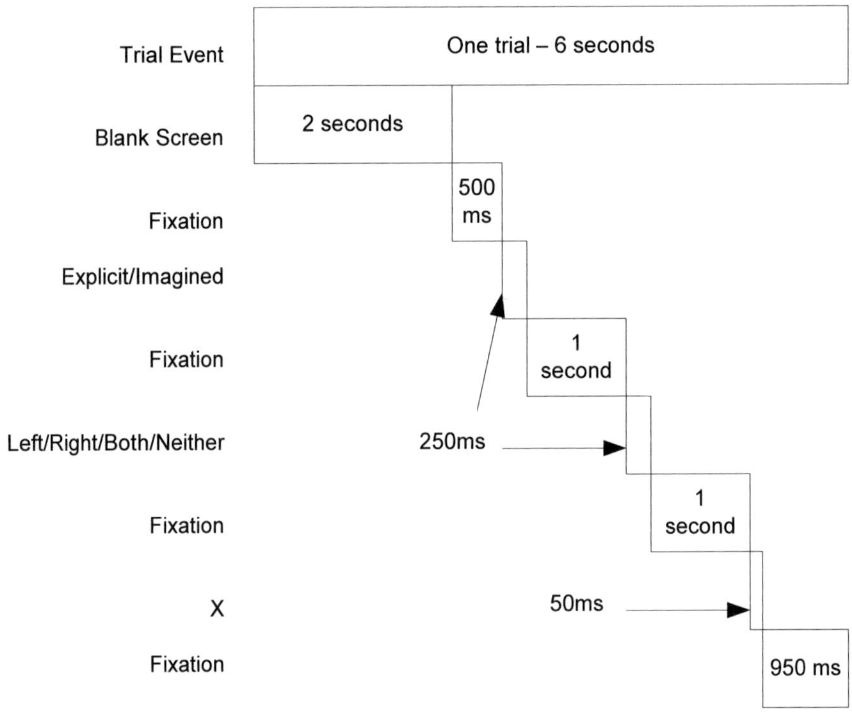

Fig. 6. Illustration of one trial recording (reproduced from http://liinc.bme.columbia.edu/EEG_DATA/EEGdescription.htm).

5.2 Experimental Setup

In order to test the BCI system, we have considered two segments from each period: A segment of 2 seconds corresponding to the blank screen, and a segment corresponding to the thinking of a movement. Only subject 1 was used in our experiments, for whom sensors coordinates (skull) were available. Ninety periods were available for this subject in the database. These were divided into 60 periods for training and 30 periods for testing. The cortical surface geometrical information was not available, however. Thus, two models have been defined for the grid. First, the spherical grid of a radius approximately equal to half of the distance between T7 and T8 of the International 10-20 system was used to represent the cortical surface. This sphere defined the grid that contains 100 points. Second, the non analytic grid defined in section 3.1 leading to approximately 120 points.

5.3 Brain Imaging Using MUSIC

Because the BCI system is based upon the calculation of neural activity on the cortical surface of the brain, it would be interesting to measure the ability of the MUSIC algorithm to detect this activity. Fig. 7 and Fig. 8 illustrate the subcorrelation coefficients for the 120 points of the non parametric grid in left action and right action. The figures also show the placement of the skull sensors (International 10-20 system). Figures were obtained using the MAP3D software. It is clear that electrical activity occurs in the same part of the cortical surface with deviation depending on the direction of the actions.

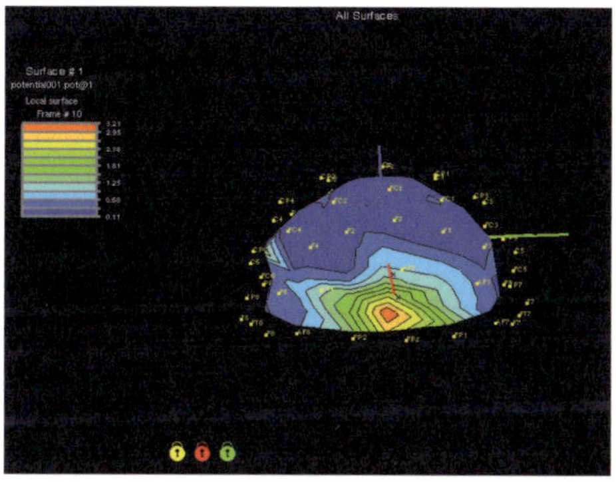

Fig. 7. Subcorrelation coefficients for left action.

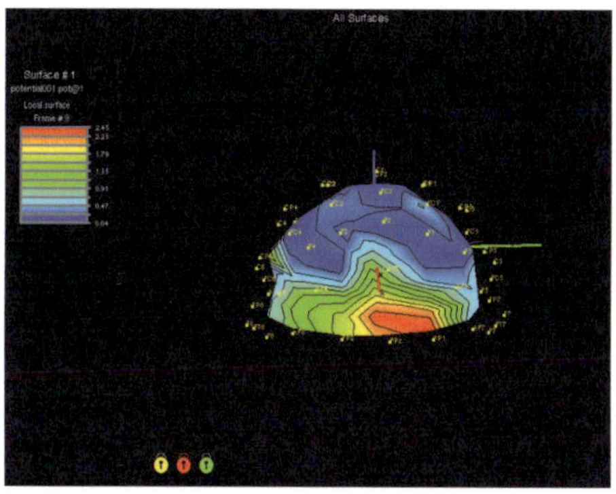

Fig. 8. Subcorrelation coefficients for right action.

5.4 MLP-Based Classifier

The first set of experiments aimed to optimize the classifier complexity, the number of cells in the hidden layer of the ANN. The analysis window on which the MUSIC algorithm is applied had a duration of 640 ms. It was assumed that the space dimension (number of dipoles) is equal to 10. The spherical grid was used in these experiments. The optimal number of hidden cells was found to be 15. One critical issue in the subspace correlation method is the dimension of the space, i.e. to determine the number of dipoles. Experiments have been conducted varying this number. Fig. 9 shows that the optimal dimension ranged between 10 and 15.

In the final set of MLP experiments, we have tried to optimize the length of the analysis window. In Fig. 10, error rates are shown for two window lengths: 640 ms and 1280 ms. The results show a better performance with the larger window. An error rate of 27% was reached.

In the last experiment with MLP classifier, the non analytic grid is used. The other parameters were fixed to what is empirically found using the spherical grid. The error rate decreased to 24%. This shows that the choice of the grid is critical.

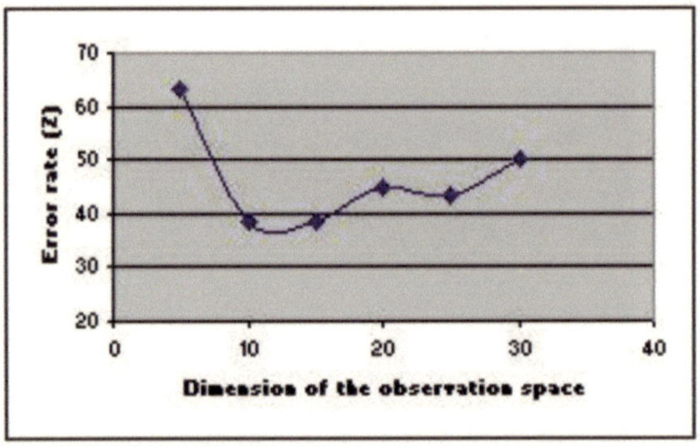

Fig. 9. Error rate function of the dimension of the observation space for MLP.

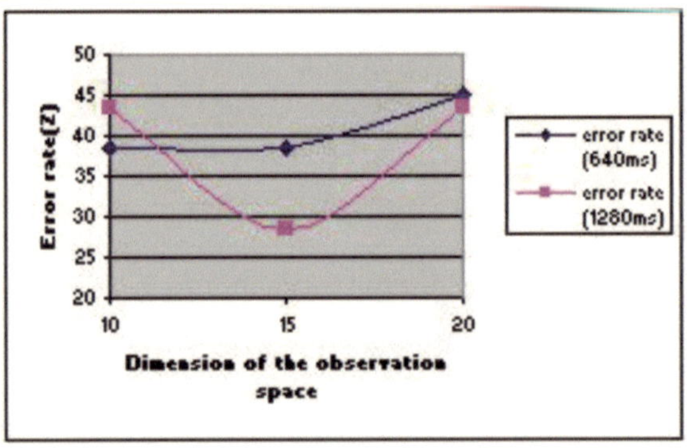

Fig. 10. Error rate function of the analysis window length: 640 ms and 1280 ms.

5.5 SVM-Based Classifier

Several kernel functions have been used: polynomial with degree 3, radial basis function, and hyperbolic tangent function. The parameters for each classifier have been optimized. Recall that the classification task is a three-class problem, the three classes being left action, right action or neither. Results are shown below in Table 1. For these experiments, features extracted on the non-parametric grid with optimal parameters found previously are used. The results demonstrate that the SVM classifier outperforms the MLP classifier.

Classifier	Error rate (%)
Artificial Neural Network MLP	24 %
SVM Polynomial Kernel	17 %
SVM Radial Basis Kernel	16.7 %
SVM Hyperbolic Tangent Kernel	20 %

Table 1. Error rates obtained with SVM classifiers compared to MLP.

In order to quantify the ability of the system to distinguish between "action" and "no action" events and between "left action" and "right action" events, experiments with a two classes-classification have been conducted. The results shown in Table 2 demonstrate that it is much easier to distinguish between "action" and "no action" classes than to determine which action has been thought. The Radial basis Kernel seems to provide the best results. These results outperform the best result obtained in (Sajda 2003), i.e. 24%.

	Error rate (%)	
Classifier	action/no action	left/right
SVM Polynomial Kernel	4%	23 %
SVM Radial Basis Kernel	4%	16.7 %
SVM Hyperbolic Tangent Kernel	4%	27 %

Table 2. SVM classification performance in a two classes- classification problems.

6. Conclusions

Brain computer interfaces have gained large interest in the last decade. Two classes of approaches are distinguished: invasive and non-invasive. While invasive approaches require the implantation of sensors in a high risk surgery, non-invasive approaches rely on advanced signal processing and pattern recognition algorithms. Those algorithms are divided into two stages: a feature extraction stage and decoding/classification stage. Classical feature extraction algorithms try to explore the time-frequency characteristics of the EEG signals (Wavelet, Filter banks) or to statistically analyze the EEG signals (PCA, ICA) in order to reduce relevant features that would help to decode the intended action. An approach proposed by (Khachab et al., 2007) consists of using a brain imaging algorithm to deduce the electrical activity on a grid defined on the cortical surface. These activations are considered to form a feature vector.

Several decoding/classification algorithms have been proposed in the literature. They take at their input the feature vectors and, based on those inputs, identify the intended action. Several machine learning algorithms have been used for this purpose. The chapter has briefly described the Artificial Neural Networks (ANN) and the Support Vector Machines (SVM).

The results obtained with a BCI system that we have developed on a reference database have shown that the use of brain imaging permits to improve the performance of the BCI. They also show that SVM classifier outperforms the ANN in all the experiments conducted.

Finally, one should notice that both the human control system (Fig. 3) and the BCI system (Fig. 1) include a feedback mechanism. However, the feedback mechanism in the BCI replaces somehow the human integrated one. This is due to the slow rate of information that can be processed by the BCI. Recent development tries to bypass the trial structure in order to overcome this problem. Important achievements have been obtained in this direction (Blankertz et al., 2006).

7. References

Anderson, C.; Stolz, E. & Shamsunder, S. (1998). Multivariate autoregressive models for classification of spontaneous Electroencephalogram during mental tasks. *IEEE Transactions on Biomedical Engineering*, Vol. 45, No 3, March 1998, 277-286, ISSN 0018-9294.

Berne, R.M.; Levy, M.N.; Koeppen, B.M. & Stanton, B.A. (1998). *Physiology, fourth edition*, Mosby Inc., ISBN: 0815109520, February 1998.

Blankertz, B.; Muller, K.-R.; Krusienski, D.J.; Schalk, G.; Wolpaw, J.R.; Schlogl, A.; Pfurtscheller, G.; Millan, Jd.R.; Schroder, M. & Birbaumer, N. (2006). The BCI competition III: validating alternative approaches to actual BCI problems. *IEEE Trans. on Neural Systems and Rehabilitation Engineering*, Vol. 14, No. 2, June 2006, 153-159, ISSN: 1534-4320.

Cristianini, N. & Shawe-Taylor, J. (2000). *An Introduction to Support Vector Machines and Other Kernel Based Learning Methods*. Cambridge University Press, ISBN: 0521780195, March 2000.

Darvishi, S. & A. Al Ani (2007). Brain-computer interface analysis using continuous wavelet transform and adaptive neuro-fuzzy classifier. *Proceedings of the International Conference on Engineering in Medicine and Biology Society* (*EMBS*), pp. 3220-3223, ISBN: 978-1-4244-0787-3, Lyon France, August 2007.

Dale, A.M. & Sereno, M.I. (1993). Improved localization of cortical activity by combining EEG and MEG with MRI cortical surface reconstruction. *Journal of Cognitive Neuroscience*, Vol. 5, 1993, 162–76.

Ebrahimi, T.; Vesin, J.M. & Garcia, G.(2003). Brain-computer interface in multimedia communication. *IEEE Signal Processing Magazine*, Vol. 20, No. 1, January 2003, 12-24, ISSN 1053-5888.

Fatourechi, M.; Mason, S.G.; Birch, G.E. & Ward, R.K. (2004). A wavelet-based approach for the extraction of the event related potentials from EEG. *Proceedings of the International Conference on Acoustic Speech and Signal Processing* (*ICASSP*), pp.737-740, ISBN: 0-7803-8484-9, Montreal-Canada, May 2004.

Garcia, G.N.; Ebrahimi, T. & Vesin, J.M. (2003). Support vector EEG classification in the fourier and time-frequency correlation domains. *Proceedings of the IEEE-EMBS First International Conference on Neural Engineering*, pp. 591-594, ISBN: 0-7803-7579-3, March 2003.

Gavit, L.; Baillet, S.; Mangin, J.F.; Pescatore, J. & Garnero. L. (2001). A multiresolution framework to MEG/EEG source imaging. *IEEE Trans. Biomedical Engineering*, Vol. 48, No. 10, October 2001, 1080-1087, ISSN: 0018-9294.

Hammon, P.S. & de Sa, V.R. (2007). Pre-Processing and meta-classification for brain-computer interfaces. *IEEE Trans. Biomedical Engineering*, Vol. 54, No. 3, March 2007, 518-525, ISSN: 0018-9294.

Hammon, P.S.; Makeig, S.; Poizner, H.; Todorov, E. & de Sa, V.R. (2008). Predicting reaching target from human EEG. *IEEE Signal Processing Magazine*, Vol. 25, No. 1, 2008, 69-77, ISSN: 1053-5888.

Hyvarinen, A. & Oja, E. (2000). Independent component analysis: Algorithms and applications. *Neural Networks*, Vol. 13, No. 4-5, 2000, 411-430, ISSN: 0893-6080.

Jakson, S.R.; Jakson, G.M. & Roberts, M. (1999). The selection and suppression of action: ERP correlates of executive control in humans. *Neuroreport*, Vol. 10, No. 4, 1999, 861-865, ISSN 0959-4965.

Jasper, H.H. The ten-twenty electrode system of the international federation. In: Internal Federation of Societies for Electroencephalography and Clinical Neurophysiology. Recommendations for the practice of clinical electroencephalography. Elsevier, Amsterdam, 1983: 3-10

Jung, T.P.; Makeig, S.; McKeown, M.J.; Bell, A.; Lee, T.W. & Sejnowski, T.J. (2001). Imaging Brain dynamics using independent component analysis. *Proceedings of the IEEE*. Vol. 89, No. 7, July 2001, 1107-1122, ISSN 0018-9219.

Kay, S.M. (1999). Modern spectral Estimation: theory and application. *Prentice Hall,* ISBN: 0130151599, Nj.

Khachab, M.; Kaakour, S. & Mokbel, C. (2007). Brain imaging and support vector machines for brain computer interface. *International Symposium on Biomedical Imaging, From Nano to Macro*, pp 1032-1035, ISBN 1-4244-0672-2, April 2007, Arlington.

Knuutila, J.E.; Ahonen, A.I.; Hamalainen, M.S.; Kajola, M.J.; Laine, P.P. & Lounasmaa, O.V. (1993). A 122-channel whole-cortex SQUID system for measuring the brain's magnetic fields. *IEEE Trans. Magnetics*, Vol. 29, No. 6, November 1993, 3315-3320, ISSN 0018-9464.

Lagerlund, T.D.; Sharbrough, F.W. & Busacker, N.E. (1997). Spatial filtering of multichannel electroencephalographic recordings through principal component analysis by singular value decomposition. *Journal Clinical Neurophysiology*, Vol. 14, No. 1, January 1997, 73-82, ISSN 0736-0258.

Michel, C.; Murray, M.; Lantz, G.; Gonzalez, S.; Spinelli, L. & Grave de Peralta, R. (2004). EEG source imaging. *Clinical Neurophysiology*. Vol. 115, No. 10, October 2004, 2195-2222, ISSN 1388-2457.

Mosher, J.C.; Lewis, P.S. & Leahy, R.M. (1992). Multiple dipole modeling and localization from spatio-temporal MEG data. *IEEE Trans. Biomedical Engineering*, Vol. 39, No. 6, June 1992, 541–557, ISSN 0018-9294.

Mosher, J.C. & Leahy. R.M. (1998). Recursive music: A framework for EEG and MEG source localization. *IEEE Trans. on Biomedical Engineering*. Vol. 45, No. 11, November 1998, 1342-1354, ISSN 0018-9294.

Mosher, J.C. & Leahy. R.M. (1999). Source localization using recursively applied and projected (rap) MUSIC. *IEEE Trans. on Signal Processing*, Vol. 47, No. 2, February 1999, 332-340, ISSN 1053-587X.

Pregenzer, M. & Pfurtscheller, G. (1999). Frequency component selection for an EEG-based brain to computer interface. *IEEE Trans. Rehabilitation Engineering*, Vol. 7, No. 4, December 1999, 413-417, ISSN 1063-6528.

Rajapakse, J.C. & Piyaratna, J. (2001). Bayesian Approach to segmentation of statistical parametric maps. *IEEE Trans. Biomedical Engineering*. Vol. 48, No. 10, October 2001, 1186-1194, ISSN 0018-9294.

Sajda, P.; Gerson, A.; Muller, K.R.; Blankertz, B. & Parra, L. (2003). A data analysis competition to evaluate machine learning algorithms for use in brain-computer interfaces. *IEEE Trans. Neural Systems and rehabilitation Engineering*, Vol. 11, No. 2, June 2003, 184-185, ISSN 1534-4320.

Sajda, P.; Muller, K-R. & Shenoy, K.V. (2008), Brain-Computer Interfaces, *IEEE Signal Processing Magazine*, Vol. 25, No. 1, January 2008, 16-17, ISSN 1053-5888.

Schmidt, R.O. (1981). A signal subspace approach to multiple emitter location and spectral estimation. PhD Thesis, *Stanford University*. 1981.

Shenoy, K.V.; Santhanam, G.; Ryu, S.I. ; Afshar, A. ; Yu, B.M.; Kalmar, R.S.; Cunningham, J.P.; Kemere, C.T.; Batista, A.P.; Churchland, M.M. & Meng, T.H. (2006). Increasing the performance of cortically-controlled protheses. *Proceedings of the International Conference on Engineering in Medicine and Biology Society* (*EMBS*), pp. 6652-6656, ISBN 1-4244-0032-5, New York, September 2006.

Vapnik, V. (1998). *Statistical Learning Theory*. Wiley, ISBN 0-471-03003-1, NY, 1998.

Veltink, P.H.; Koopman, H.F.J.M.; van der Helm, F.C.T. & Nene, A.V. (2001). Biomechatronics-assisting the impaired motor system. *Archives of physiology and Biochemistry*, Vol. 109, No. 1, 2001, 1-9.

Müller, K-R. & Blankertz, B. (2006). Toward non-invasive brain-computer interfaces. *IEEE Signal Processing Magazine*, Vol. 128, No. 1, September 2006, 125-128, ISSN 1053-5888.

Vorobyov, S. & Cichoki, A. (2002). Blind noise reduction for multisensory signals using ICA and subspace filtering, with application to EEG analysis. *Biological Cybernetics*. Vol. 86, No. 4, April 2002, 293-303, ISSN 0340-1200.

Westbrook. G.L. (2000). Seizures and epilepsy. In: *Principles of Neural Science*. Kandel, E.R., Schwartz, J.H., and Jessel, T.M., Editors. Fourth edition., 910-935, McGraw Hill, ISBN 0838577016.

Wolpaw, J.R.; Birbaumer, N.; McFarland, D.J.; Pfurtscheller, G. & Vaughan, T. (2002). Brain-computer interfaces for communication and control. *Clinical Neurophysiology*, Vol. 113, No. 6, June 2002, 767-791, ISSN 1388-2457.

Xu, B.; Song, A. & Wu, J. (2007). Algorithm of imagined left-right hand movement classification based on wavelet transform and AR parameter model. *Proceedings of the International Conference on Bioinformatics and Biomedical Engineering* (*ICBBE*), pp. 539-542, ISBN 1-4244-1120-3, Wuhan, July 2007.

http://software.sci.utah.edu/map3d.

4

Texture Analysis Methods for Medical Image Characterisation

William Henry Nailon
Department of Oncology Physics, Edinburgh Cancer Centre & School of Engineering, University of Edinburgh, United Kingdom

1. Introduction

Texture analysis refers to the branch of imaging science that is concerned with the description of characteristic image properties by textural features. However, there is no universally agreed-upon definition of what image texture is and in general different researchers use different definitions depending upon the particular area of application (Tuceryan & Jain, 1998). In this chapter texture is defined as the spatial variation of pixel intensities, which is a definition that is widely used and accepted in the field. The main image processing disciplines in which texture analysis techniques are used are classification, segmentation and synthesis. In image classification the goal is to classify different images or image regions into distinct groups (Pietikainen, 2000). Texture analysis methods are well suited to this because they provide unique information on the texture, or spatial variation of pixels, of the region where they are applied. In image segmentation problems the aim is to establish boundaries between different image regions (Mirmehdi et al., 2008). By applying texture analysis methods to an image, and determining the precise location where texture feature values change significantly, boundaries between regions can be established. Synthesising image texture is important in three-dimensional (3D) computer graphics applications where the goal is to generate highly complex and realistic looking surfaces. Fractals have proven to be a mathematically elegant means of generating textured surfaces through the iteration of concise equations (Pentland, 1984). Conversely the ability to accurately represent a textured surface by a concise set of fractal equations has led to significant advances in image compression applications using fractal methods (Distani et al., 2006)

An example of image classification is presented in Fig. 1 in which it is possible to uniquely identify the two different textures (left, grass; right, water) by eye. In Fig. 2 the image on the left is a composite image formed from eight Brodatz textures, all of which are represented in approximately equal proportions. The right image is a grey-level texture map showing the ideal segmentation of the textures (Weber, 2004).

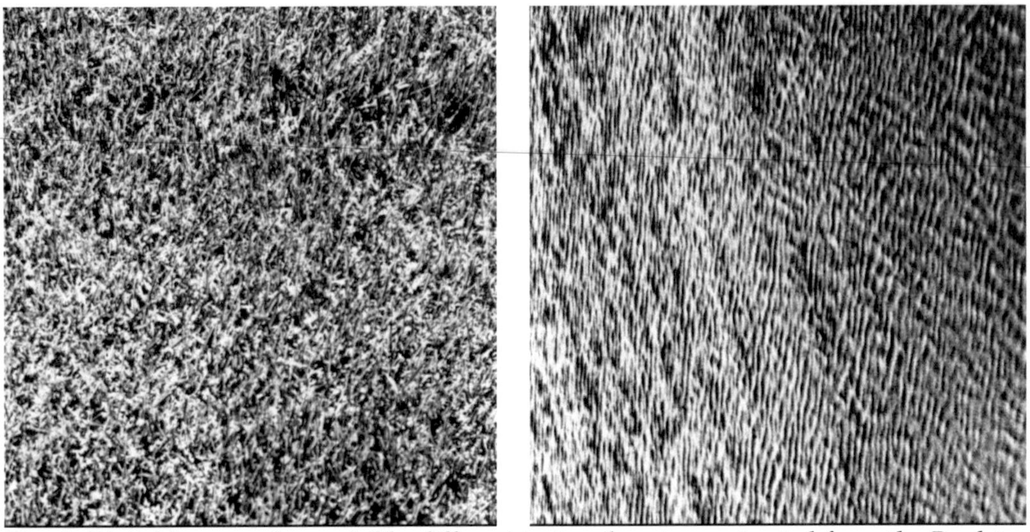

Fig. 1. Digital images of two visibly different textured regions extracted from the Brodatz texture database (Brodatz, 1966). Left, image of grass (1.2.01, D9 H.E.). Right, image of water (1.2.08, D38 H.E.) (Weber, 2004).

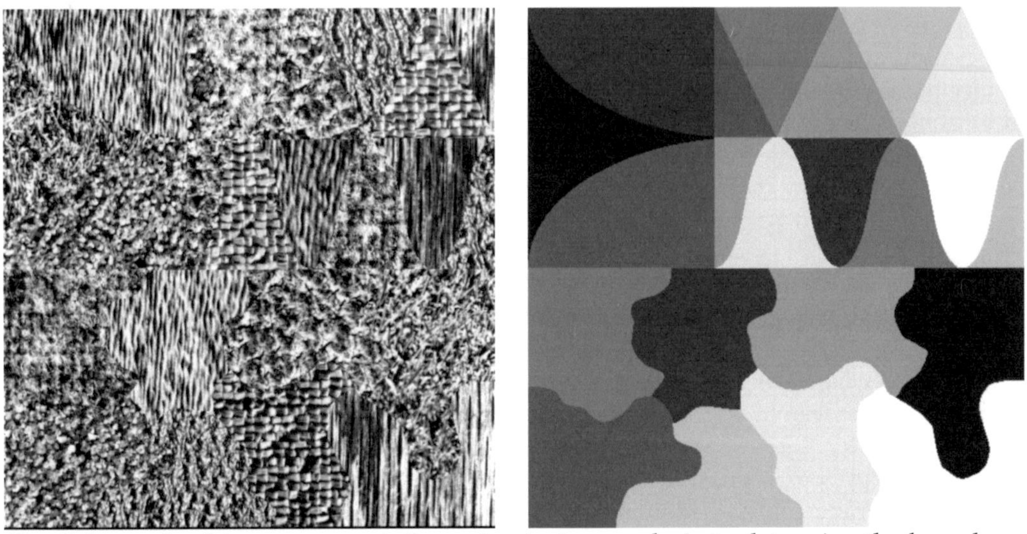

Fig. 2. Example of image segmentation using texture analysis to determine the boundary between distinct regions of texture. Left, mosaic image of eight Brodatz textures represented in approximately equal proportions. Right, grey-level texture map showing the ideal segmentation of the textures (Weber, 2004).

2. The Visual Perception of Texture

Much of our understanding of machine vision algorithms is a result of attempts to overcome the failings of the human visual system to detect certain textured patterns. This understanding has proven vital in evaluating and comparing the performance of human vision against machine-based texture analysis approaches. Julesz, an experimental psychologist, was an early pioneer in the visual perception of texture (Julesz, 1975). He was responsible for establishing authoritative data on the performance of the human vision system at discriminating certain classes of texture. He verified that discriminating between two image textures depends largely upon the difference in the second-order statistics of the textures. That is, for two textures with identical second-order statistics a deliberate amount of effort is required to discriminate between them. In contrast little effort is required when the second-order statistics of the textures are different. However, this observation does not extend to textures that differ in third- or higher-order statistics, which are not readily discriminated by eye (Julesz, 1975). This is illustrated in Fig. 3 in which each of the main textured images (left and right) has a smaller area of similar, but subtly different, texture embedded within it. In the image on the left both the main and embedded areas have identical first-order statistics, however, their second-order statistics are different making it straightforward to discriminate both regions. In the image on the right both textures have identical first- and second-order statistics and therefore it is only after careful scrutiny that the different textured regions become visible.

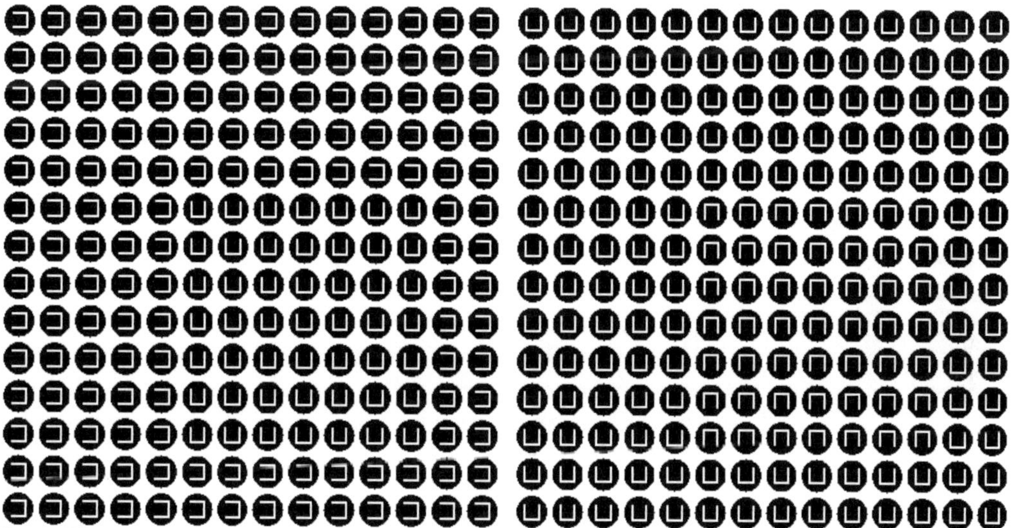

Fig. 3. The images on the left and right have a main area of texture embedded within which is a smaller area of similar, but subtly different, texture. In the left image both textures have the same first-order statistics and different second-order statistics, which makes it straightforward for an observer to distinguish between them. In the image on the right both textures have identical first- and second-order statistics and hence only after careful scrutiny are the different patterns visible (Julesz, 1975).

Although our understanding of the cognitive process of human vision is constantly expanding much has been learned from experiments in the visual perception of digital image information (Bruce et al, 2003). Such work is vital, particularly in medical imaging where the misinterpretation of image information can have a serious impact on health (ICRU, 1999). This is particularly apparent in radiotherapy, the treatment of cancer by ionising radiation, where the aim is to deliver as high a radiation dose as possible to diseased tissue whilst limiting the radiation dose to healthy tissue. Delineation of the tumour volume is based primarily on visual assessment of computerised tomographic (CT) and magnetic resonance (MR) image data by a radiation oncologist. Accurately defining the tumour, and potential areas of tumour involvement, on CT and MR data is a complex image interpretation process requiring considerable clinical experience. As a result significant inter- and intra-clinician variability has been reported in the contouring of tumours of the lung, prostate, brain and oesophagus (Weltens et al., 2001; Steenbakkers et al., 2005). This variability has been shown to be significant and heavily correlated with the digital imaging modality used and the image settings applied during the assessment.

Texture analysis is presented here as a useful computational method for discriminating between pathologically different regions on medical images because it has been proven to perform better than human eyesight at discriminating certain classes of texture (Julesz, 1975). Section 3 presents statistical texture analysis through first-, second-, and higher-order techniques. Section 4 considers the use of fractal methods for characterising image texture through the box-counting and Korcak techniques. In section 5 methods are presented for improving the overall efficiency of the texture analysis approach. These are feature selection, reduction and classification. Section 6 presents two case studies, which demonstrate the use of these approaches in practical biomedical imaging.

3. Statistical Approaches for Texture Analysis

To examine an image using texture analysis the image is treated as a 3D textured surface. This is illustrated in Fig. 4 which shows the textured intensity surface representation of a two-dimensional (2D) medical image. In first-order statistical texture analysis, information on texture is extracted from the histogram of image intensity. This approach measures the frequency of a particular grey-level at a random image position and does not take into account correlations, or co-occurrences, between pixels. In second-order statistical texture analysis, information on texture is based on the probability of finding a pair of grey-levels at random distances and orientations over an entire image. Extension to higher-order statistics involves increasing the number of variables studied.

Many conventional approaches used to study texture have concentrated on using 2D techniques to compute features relating to image texture. This traditional approach has been used extensively to describe different image textures by unique features and has found application in many disparate fields such as: discrimination of terrain from aerial photographs (Conners & Harlow, 1980); in vitro classification of tissue from intravascular ultrasound (Nailon, 1997); identification of prion protein distribution in cases of Creutzfeld-Jakob disease (CJD) (Nailon & Ironside, 2000); classification of pulmonary emphysema from lung on high-resolution CT images (Uppaluri et al., 1997; Xu et al., 2004; Xu et al., 2006); and identifying normal and cancerous pathology (Karahaliou et al., 2008, Zhou et al., 2007; Yu et a., 2009). Higher-order approaches have been used to localise thrombotic tissue in the aorta (Podda, 2005) and to determine if functional vascular information found in dynamic MR sequences exists on anatomical MR sequences (Winzenrieth, 2006). Extension of these approaches to 3D is continuing to develop within the machine vision community. Several authors have reported the application of 2D texture analysis methods on a slice-by-slice basis through volumetric data, however, it has been reported that with this approach information may be lost (Kovalev et al., 2001; Kurani et al., 2004). Findings reported by Xu et al., on the use of 3D textural features for discriminating between smoking related lung pathology, demonstrate the power of this approach for this particular application (Xu et al., 2006). Kovalev et al., showed that an extended 3D co-occurrence matrix approach can be used for the classification and segmentation of diffuse brain lesions on MR image data (Kovalev et al., 2001). Texture analysis has also been used to identify unique pathology on multi-modality images of cancer patients. Using the local binary operator to analyse the weak underlying textures found in transrectal ultrasound images of the prostate, Kachouie and Fieguth demonstrated that the approach was suitable for segmentation of the prostate (Kachouie & Fieguth, 2007). In another cancer-related study of 48 normal images and 58 cancer images of the colon, Esgiar et al., demonstrated that by adding a fractal feature to traditional statistical features the sensitivity of the classification improved (Esgiar et al., 2002).

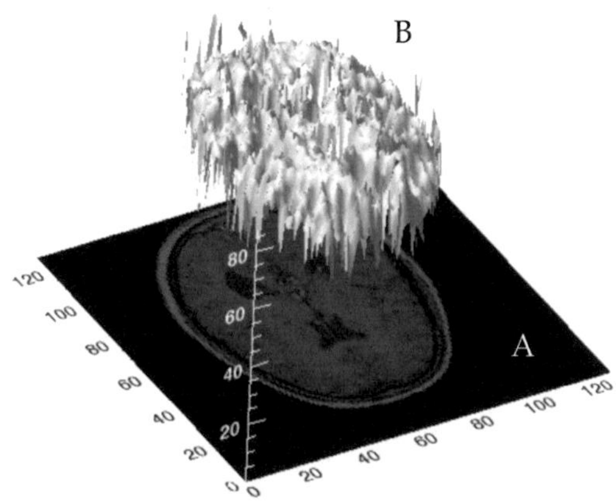

Fig. 4. Three-dimensional textured intensity surface representation of a medical image. **A**: Two-dimensional MR image of the brain. **B**: Pixel values of the MR image plotted on the vertical axis to produce a 3D textured surface.

With the proliferation of 3D medical image data of near isotropic quality there is an increasing demand for artificial intelligence methods capable of deriving quantitative measures relating to distinct pathology. The remaining sections of this chapter provide a review of statistical and fractal texture analysis approaches in the context of medical imaging and provide comprehensive real-world examples, in the form of two case studies, on the use of these approaches in clinical practice. In case study 1 texture analysis is presented as a means of classifying distinct regions in cancer images, which could be developed further towards automatic classification. In case study 2 texture analysis is presented as an objective means of identifying the different patterns of prion protein found in variant CJD (vCJD) and sporadic CJD. Two contrasting methods are presented in the case studies for evaluating the performance of the texture analysis methodologies.

3.1 First-Order Statistical Texture Analysis

First-order texture analysis measures use the image histogram, or pixel occurrence probability, to calculate texture. The main advantage of this approach is its simplicity through the use of standard descriptors (e.g. mean and variance) to characterise the data (Press, 1998). However, the power of the approach for discriminating between unique textures is limited in certain applications because the method does not consider the spatial relationship, and correlation, between pixels. For any surface, or image, grey-levels are in the range $0 \le i \le N_g - 1$, where N_g is the total number of distinct grey-levels. If $N(i)$ is the number of pixels with intensity i and M is the total number of pixels in an image, it follows that the histogram, or pixel occurrence probability, is given by,

$$P(i) = \frac{N(i)}{M}. \tag{1}$$

In general seven features commonly used to describe the properties of the image histogram, and therefore image texture, are computed. These are: mean; variance; coarseness; skewness; kurtosis; energy; and entropy.

3.2 Second-Order Statistical Texture Analysis

The human visual system cannot discriminate between texture pairs with matching second-order statistics (see Fig. 3) (Julesz, 1975). The first machine-vision framework for calculating second-order or pixel co-occurrence texture information was developed for analysing aerial photography images (Haralick et al., 1973). In this technique pixel co-occurrence matrices, which are commonly referred to as grey-tone spatial dependence matrices (GTSDM), are computed. The entries in a GTSDM are the probability of finding a pixel with grey-level i at a distance d and angle α from a pixel with a grey-level j. This may be written more formally as $P(i, j : d, \alpha)$. An essential component of this framework is that each pixel has eight nearest-neighbours connected to it, except at the periphery. As a result four GTSDMs are required to describe the texture content in the horizontal $(P_H = 0^0)$, vertical $(P_V = 90^0)$ right- $(P_{RD} = 45^0)$ and left-diagonal $(P_{LD} = 135^0)$ directions. This is illustrated in Fig. 5.

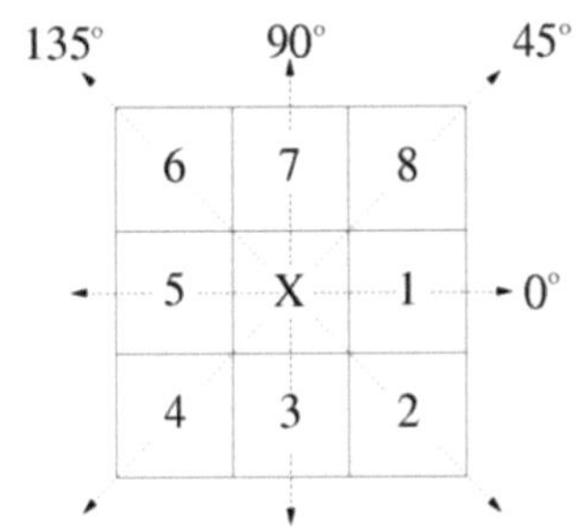

Fig. 5. Eight nearest-neighbour pixels used in the GTSDM framework to describe pixel connectivity. Cells 1 and 5 show the horizontal (P_H), 4 and 8 the right-diagonal (P_{RD}), 3 and 7 the vertical (P_V) and 2 and 6 the left-diagonal (P_{LD}) nearest-neighbours.

An example of the calculation of a horizontal co-occurrence matrix (P_H) on a 4×4 image containing four unique grey-levels is shown in Fig. 6. A complete representation of image texture is contained in the co-occurrence matrices calculated in the four directions. Extracting information from these matrices using textural features, which are sensitive to specific elements of texture, provides unique information on the structure of the texture being investigated. Haralick et al., proposed a set of 14 local features specifically designed for this purpose (Haralick et al., 1973). In practice the information provided by certain features may be highly correlated or of limited practical use. A feature selection strategy is therefore useful with this approach to take account of redundant, or irrelevant, information. This is discussed in more detail in section 5. It is also interesting to note that prior to any processing the GTSDMs, which are symmetric, can provide some useful information on the characteristics of the image being studied. For example, the co-occurrence matrix entries for a coarse texture will be heavily focused along the diagonals relative to the distance d between the pixels studied.

0	2	2	2
0	3	2	2
1	2	2	2
3	0	3	0

(P_H)

0^0 (Grey-Level)	Grey-Level 0	1	2	3
0	0	0	1	4
1	0	0	1	0
2	1	1	10	1
3	4	0	1	0

Fig. 6. Simple example demonstrating the formation of a co-occurrence matrix from an image. Left, 4×4 image with four unique grey-levels. Right, the resulting horizontal co-occurrence matrix (P_H).

To illustrate the computational requirements of this framework, three of the 14 features proposed by Haralick et al., (Haralick et al., 1973) are presented in equations 2 to 4.

Angular second moment,

$$f_1 = \sum_{i=1}^{N_q}\sum_{j=1}^{N_q} p'(i,j)^2. \tag{2}$$

Contrast,

$$f_2 = \sum_{i=0}^{Nq-1} n^2 \left[\sum_{i=1}^{Nq}\sum_{j=1}^{Nq} p'(i,j) \right]_{i-j=n} . \tag{3}$$

Correlation,

$$f_3 = \sum_{i=1}^{N_q}\sum_{j=1}^{N_q} \frac{(i-\mu_x)(j-\mu_y)p'(i,j)}{\sigma_x\sigma_y}, \tag{4}$$

where, N_q is the number of distinct grey-levels in the input and μ_x, μ_y, σ_x and σ_y are the means and standard deviations of $p'(i,j)$. Throughout, $p'(i,j) = P(i,j)/R$, where $P(i,j)$ is the average of $(P_H + P_V + P_{LD} + P_{RD})$ and R is the maximum number of resolution cells in a GTSDM.

3.3 Higher-Order Statistical Texture Analysis

The grey-level run length method (GLRLM) is based on the analysis of higher-order statistical information (Galloway, 1975). In this approach GLRLMs contain information on the run of a particular grey-level, or grey-level range, in a particular direction. The number of pixels contained within the run is the run-length. A coarse texture will therefore be dominated by relatively long runs whereas a fine texture will be populated by much shorter runs. The number of runs r' with gray-level i, or lying within a grey-level range i, of run-length j in a direction α is denoted by $R(\alpha) = [r'(i,j \mid \alpha)]$. This is analogous to the GTSDM technique (Haralick et al., 1973) as four GTRLMs are commonly used to describe texture runs in the directions ($0^0, 45^0, 90^0$ and 135^0) on linearly adjacent pixels. An example of the calculation of a horizontal GLRLM is shown in Fig. 7.

0	1	2	2
0	3	2	2
1	2	2	2
3	0	3	0

		Run-Length			
	0^0	1	2	3	4
Grey-Level	0	4	0	0	0
	1	2	0	0	0
	2	0	2	1	0
	3	3	0	0	0

Fig. 7. Simple example demonstrating the formation of a GLRLM. Left, 4×4 image with four unique grey-levels. Right, the resulting GLRLM in the direction 0^0.

A set of seven numerical texture measures are computed from the GTRLMs. Three of these measures are presented here to illustrate the computation of feature information using this framework.

Short Run Emphasis,

$$f_{SR} = \frac{1}{T_R} \sum_{i=0}^{N_g - 1} \sum_{j=1}^{N_r} \frac{r'(i,j \mid \alpha)}{j^2}. \tag{5}$$

Long Run Emphasis,

$$f_{LR} = \frac{1}{T_R} \sum_{i=0}^{N_g - 1} \sum_{j=1}^{N_r} j^2 r'(i,j \mid \alpha). \tag{6}$$

Grey-Level Distribution,

$$f_{GD} = \frac{1}{T_R} \sum_{i=0}^{N_g-1} \left[\sum_{j=1}^{N_r} r'(i,j \mid \alpha) \right]^2, \tag{7}$$

where N_g is the maximum number of grey-levels, N_r is the number of different run lengths in the matrix and,

$$T_R = \sum_{i=0}^{N_g-1} \sum_{j=1}^{N_r} r'(i,j \mid \alpha). \tag{8}$$

T_R serves as a normalising factor in each of the run length equations.

3.4 Fourier Power Spectrum

Two-dimensional transforms have been used extensively in image processing to tackle problems such as image description and enhancement (Pratt, 1978). Of these, the Fourier transform is one of the most widely used (Gonzalez and Woods, 2001). Fourier analysis can be used to study the properties of textured scenes, for example the power spectrum reveals information on the coarseness/fineness (periodicity) and directionality of a texture. Texture directionality is preserved in the power spectrum because it allows directional and non-directional components of the texture to be distinguished (Bajscy, 1973). These observations have given rise to two powerful approaches for extracting texture primitives from the Fourier power spectrum, namely, ring and wedge filters. Working from the origin of the power spectrum the coarseness/fineness is measured between rings of inner radius r_1 and r_2. The size of the rings can be varied according to the application. The directionality of the texture is found by measuring the average power over wedge-shaped regions centred at the origin of the power spectrum. The size of the wedge $\phi_w = \phi_1 - \phi_2$ depends upon the application. Fig. 8 illustrates the extraction of ring and wedge filters from the Fourier power spectrum of a 32×32 test image consisting of black pixels everywhere except for a 3×3 region of white pixels centred at the origin.

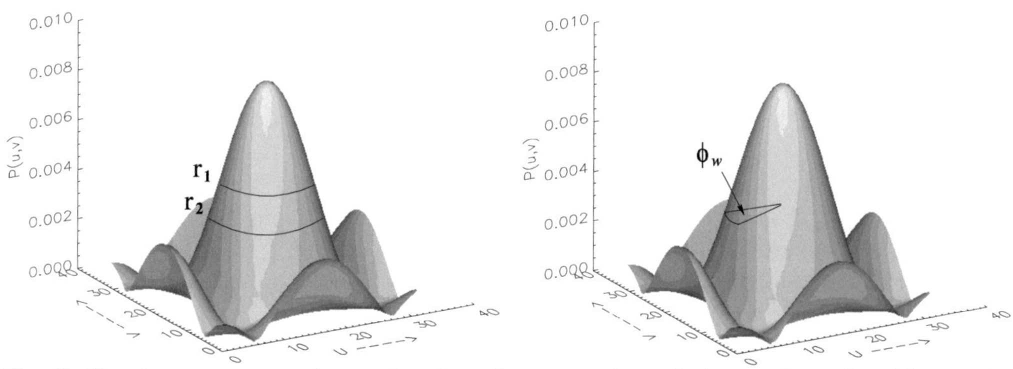

Fig. 8. Fourier power spectrum showing the extraction of ring and wedge filters. The spectrum was generated on a 32×32 test image consisting of black pixels everywhere except for a 3×3 region of white pixels centred at the origin.

In image analysis the Fourier transform $F(u,v)$ is considered in its discrete form and the power spectrum $P(u,v)$ is calculated from,

$$P(u,v)=|F(u,v)|^2. \tag{9}$$

The average power contained in a ring centred at the origin with inner and outer radii r_1 and r_2 respectively, is given by the summation of the contributions along the direction ϕ ,

$$P(r)=2\sum_{\phi=0}^{\pi} P(r,\phi). \tag{10}$$

The contribution from a wedge of size ϕ_w is found from summation of the radial components within the wedge boundaries. That is,

$$P(\phi_w)=\sum_{r=0}^{n/2} P(r,\phi), \tag{11}$$

where n is the window size.

4. Fractal Texture Analysis

Until the introduction of fractals it was difficult to accurately describe, mathematically, complex real-world shapes such as mountains, coastlines, trees and clouds (Mandelbrot, 1977). Fractals provide a succinct and accurate method for describing natural objects that would previously have been described by spheres, cylinders and cubes. However, these descriptors are smooth, which makes modelling irregular natural scenes, or surfaces, very difficult. The popularity of fractals has grown considerably over the past three decades since the term was first coined by Mandelbrot to describe structures too complex for Euclidean geometry to describe by a single measure (Mandelbrot, 1977). The fractal dimension describes the degree of irregularity or texture of a surface. With this approach rougher, or more irregular, structures have a greater fractal dimension (Feder, 1988; Peitgen & Saupe, 1988; Peitgen et al., 1992).

The property of self-similarity is one of the central concepts of fractal geometry (Turcotte, 1997). An object is self-similar if it can be decomposed into smaller copies of itself. This fundamental property leads to the classification of fractals into two distinct groups, random and deterministic. A good example of self-similarity is exhibited by an aerial image of an irregular coastline structure that has the same appearance within a range of magnification factors. At each magnification the coastline will not look exactly the same but only similar. This particular feature is common to many classes of real-life random fractals, which are not exactly self-similar. These are referred to as being statistically self-similar. In contrast, objects that do not change their appearance when viewed under arbitrary magnification are termed strictly self-similar. These are termed deterministic fractals due to their consistency over a range of magnification scales. The fractal dimension describes the disorder of an object numerically, which in a sense is similar to the description of objects using standard Euclidean geometry. That is, the higher the dimension the more complicated the object. However, fractal descriptors allow the description of objects by non-integer dimensions.

A variety of techniques are used to estimate the fractal dimension of objects which, despite providing the same measure, can produce different fractal dimension values for analysis of the same object. This is due to the unique mechanism used by each technique to find the fractal dimension (Peitgen et al., 1992; Turcotte, 1997). Two approaches commonly used to calculate the fractal dimension of an image are discussed. The first is the box-counting approach (Peitgen et al., 1992). The second, which treats the input as a textured surface by plotting the intensity at each x and y position in the z plane, calculates the fractal dimension using the Korcak method (Russ, 1994).

4.1 Fractal Dimension from Box-Counting

The box-counting dimension is closely related to the concept of self-similarity where a structure is sub-divided into smaller elements, each a smaller replica of the original structure. This sub-division characterises the structure by a self-similarity, or fractal, dimension and is a useful tool for characterising apparently random structures. This approach has been adopted in a variety of applications, for example in the characterisation of high resolution satellite images (Yu et al., 2007) and in the detection of cracks in CT images of wood (Li & Qi, 2007). The box-counting dimension D_b of any bounded subset of A in $\mathbf{R}^n$, which is a set in Euclidean space, may be formally defined as follows (Stoyan & Stoyan, 1994; Peitgen & Saupe, 1988). Let $N_r(A)$ be the smallest number of sets of r that cover A. Then,

$$D_b(A) = \lim_{r \to 0} \frac{\log N_r(A)}{\log(1/r)}, \tag{12}$$

provided that the limit exists. Subdividing $\mathbf{R}^n$ into a lattice of grid size $r \times r$ where r is continually reduced, it follows that $N_r'(A)$ is the number of grid elements that intersect A and $D_b(A)$ is,

$$D_b(A) = \lim_{r \to 0} \frac{\log N_r'(A)}{\log(1/r)}, \tag{13}$$

provided that the limit exists. This implies that the box counting dimension $D_b(A)$ and $N_r(A)$ are related by the following power law relation,

$$N_r(A) = \frac{1}{r^{D_b(A)}}. \tag{14}$$

Proof of this relation can be obtained by taking logs of both sides of equation (14) and rearranging to form equation (15),

$$\log N_r(A) = D_b(A)\log(1/r). \tag{15}$$

From equation (15) it is possible to make an analogy to the equation of a straight line, $y = mx + c$, where m is the slope of the line and c is the y intersect. The box-counting dimension is implemented by placing a bounded set A, in the form of a medical image, on to a grid formed from boxes of size $r \times r$. Grid boxes containing some of the structure, which in the case of a medical image is represented by the grey-levels within a certain range, are next counted. The total number of boxes in the grid that contain some of the structure is $N_r(A)$. The algorithm continues by altering r to progressively smaller sizes and counting $N_r(A)$. The slope of the line fitted through the plot of $\log(1/r)$ against $\log(N_r(A)$ is the fractal, or box-counting, dimension of the medical image region under investigation.

4.2 Korcak Fractal Analysis

This approach uses the idea of a cross-section, or zeroset, through the surface or image to determine the fractal dimension (Russ, 1994). It is implemented by passing a horizontal plane through a 3 D surface in a vertical direction to produce an intersection profile. The points of the surface that lie above the horizontal plane are commonly referred to as islands and the remaining areas of the plane are lakes. This is equivalent to applying a threshold and measuring the area of the islands and lakes that lie above or below the surface. This is illustrated in Fig. 9 which shows the result of repeated thresholding on an image of the cerebellum for a case of vCJD. A log-log plot of the number of islands, or lakes, whose area exceeds A is fitted to a straight line (see Fig. 10). The slope of this line is used to calculate the fractal dimension. This approach is termed the Korcak method (Russ, 1994).

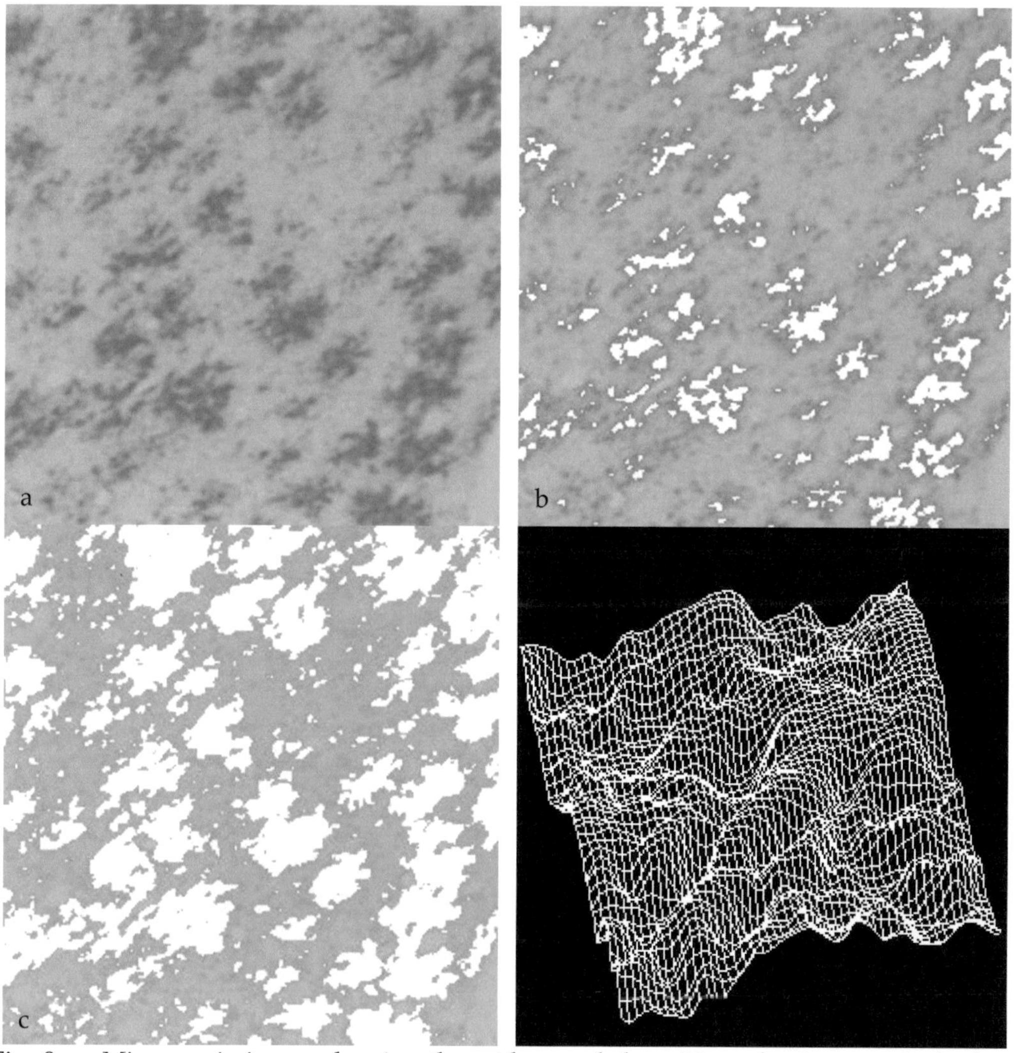

Fig. 9. **a**: Microscopic image showing the widespread deposition of prion protein in the cerebellum of a vCJD case. **b** and **c**: The result of repeated grey-level thresholding. **d**: The image surface cut by a plane or zeroset. Repeating the thresholding at many levels and constructing a Korcak plot of the cumulative number of islands provides a measure of the fractal dimension.

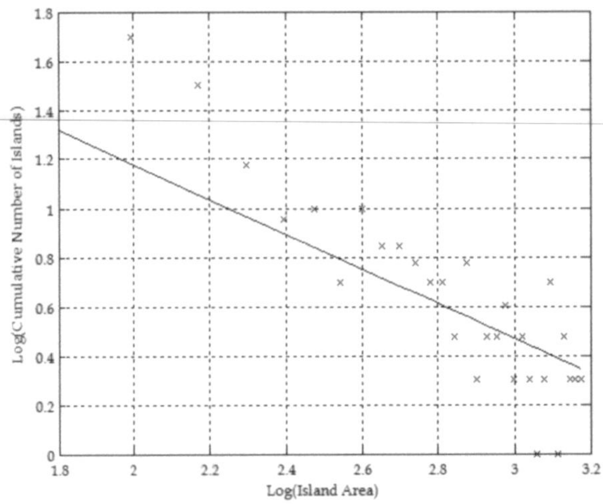

Fig. 10. Plot of fractal island area against cumulative number of islands acquired within the area. The slope of the straight line plotted through the data is used to determine the fractal dimension.

5. Feature Selection, Reduction and Classification

The texture analysis approaches presented in the preceding sections calculate features that describe properties of the image, or region, being studied. This information is next used in a pattern recognition system to classify the objects, or texture patterns of interest, into an appropriate number of categories or classes (Therrien, 1989). However, some of the features calculated may be highly correlated and some may contain irrelevant information. Feature selection is used to select a subset of features $\boldsymbol{s}_p$ from a given set of $\boldsymbol{p}$ features such that $\boldsymbol{s}_p \leq \boldsymbol{p}$ and there is no significant degradation in the performance of the classification system (Therrien, 1989; Zongker & Jain, 1996; Stearns, 1976). The reduction of the feature set reduces the dimensionality of the classification problem and in some cases can increase the performance of the classification accuracy due to finite sample size effects (Jain & Chandrasekaran, 1982). Two powerful methods for reducing the number of features are presented. These are the sequential forward search (SFS) algorithm and its backward counterpart the sequential backward search (SBS) algorithm (Devijver & Kittler, 1982). The pattern recognition system must also be capable of partitioning, or clustering, the reduced feature set into classes of similar observations. The *K*-means algorithm belongs to the collection of multivariate methods used for classifying, or clustering, data and is presented because of its general applicability in classification problems (Therrien, 1989).

5.1 Feature Selection Using the Sequential Forward Search Algorithm

The SFS algorithm is a bottom-up strategy for removing redundant or irrelevant features from the feature matrix (Devijver & Kittler, 1982). At each successive iteration the feature that produces the largest value of the selection criterion function *J* is added to the current feature set. Given a set of candidate features $Y \in \boldsymbol{R}$, a subset $X \in \boldsymbol{R}$ is selected without significant degradation to the classification system (Jain & Zongker, 1997). The best subset X,

$$X = \{x_i \mid i = 1,2,\ldots,d, \quad x_i = Y\}, \tag{16}$$

of d features where $(d \leq D)$ is selected from the set,

$$Y = \{y_1 \mid j = 1,2,\ldots,D\}, \tag{17}$$

by optimising the criterion function J, chosen here to be the estimated minimum probability of error. For the set of measurements taken from Y, ideally the probability of correct classification (ξ), with respect to any other combination, is given by,

$$\Xi = \{\xi_i \mid i = 1,2,\ldots,d\}. \tag{18}$$

It follows that the minimum probability of error for the space spanned by ξ, for each class ω_i is defined as,

$$E(\Xi) = \int [1 - \max(P(\omega_i \mid \xi))] p(\xi) d(\xi), \tag{19}$$

and the desired criterion function,

$$J(X) = \min(E(\Xi)). \tag{20}$$

One of the disadvantages of the SFS approach is that it may suffer from nesting. That is, because features selected and included in the feature subset cannot be removed, already selected features determine the course of the remaining selection process. This has noticeable hazards since after further iterations a feature may become superfluous. Another limitation of the SFS approach is that in the case of two feature variables, which alone provide little discrimination but together are very effective, the SFS approach may never detect this combination. To overcome this problem it is useful to start with a full set of available features and eliminate them one at a time. This is the method adopted by the SBS approach described in section 5.2.

5.2 Feature Selection Using the Sequential Backward Search Algorithm

The SBS is a top down approach, which starts with the complete feature set and removes one feature at each successive iteration (Devijver & Kittler, 1982). The feature that is chosen to be removed is the feature that results in the smallest reduction in the value of the selection criterion function when it is removed. In general, the SBS algorithm requires more computation than the SFS algorithm because initially it considers the number of features in the complete set as forming the subset. Although the SBS overcomes some of the difficulties of the SFS approach the resulting feature subset is not guaranteed to be optimal. Furthermore, like its counterpart the SBS algorithm suffers from nesting because once a feature is selected it cannot be disregarded. Implementation of the SBS approach is analogous to the SFS approach detailed in section 5.1. The SBS algorithm is computationally more expensive than the SFS algorithm, however, their performance is comparable. Despite the shortcomings of the SFS and SBS techniques they are powerful techniques for reducing the feature set of real-world pattern recognition problems (Nouza, 1995).

5.3 Classification Using the *K*-means Algorithm

The general clustering problem is one of identifying clusters, or classes, of similar points. For the specific problem presented in this chapter this would involve clustering the features calculated on a specific image region into a unique cluster. The number of classes may be known or unknown depending on the particular problem. The *K*-means algorithm belongs to the collection of multivariate methods used for clustering data (Therrien, 1989; Hartigan, 1975; Duda et al., 2001). The algorithm starts with a partition of the observations into clusters. At each step the algorithm moves a case from one cluster to another if the move will increase the overall similarity within clusters. The algorithm ceases when the similarity within clusters can no longer be increased.

Assuming that the number of clusters N_c is known in advance the *K*-means technique may be defined by the following three stages.

Stage 1 – *Initialisation*: For the set of observations $\boldsymbol{Y} = \{y_1, y_2 \ldots, y_N\}$ to be classified into the set of classes $\Omega = \{\omega_1, \omega_2, \ldots, \omega_{Nc}\}$, the algorithm starts with an arbitrary partition of the observations into N_c clusters and computes the mean vector of each cluster $(\mu_1, \mu_2, \ldots \mu_{Nc})$ using the Euclidean distance $\|\boldsymbol{y}_i - \boldsymbol{\mu}_k\|^2$ where $\boldsymbol{\mu}_k$ is the sample mean of the kth cluster.

Stage 2 - *Nearest Mean*: Assign each observation in $\boldsymbol{Y}$ to the cluster with the closest mean.

Stage 3 - *Update and Repeat*: Update the mean vector for each cluster and repeat *Stage 2* until the result produces no significant change in the cluster means.

6. Biomedical Image Analysis Case Studies

Two case studies are presented to demonstrate the practical application of the texture analysis methods discussed in the previous sections. In the first, a texture analysis approach was used to classify regions of distinct pathology on CT images acquired on eight bladder cancer patients. In the second, texture analysis was used to study the distribution of abnormal prion protein found in the molecular layer of the cerebellum of cases of vCJD and sporadic CJD.

6.1 Case Study 1 - Texture Analysis of Radiotherapy Planning Target Volumes

The goal of radiotherapy, the treatment of cancer with ionising radiation, is to deliver as high a dose of radiation as possible to diseased tissue whilst sparing healthy tissue. In curative (radical) radiotherapy planning, delineation of the gross tumour volume (GTV) is primarily based on visual assessment of CT images by a radiation oncologist (Meyer, 2007). The accuracy therefore of the GTV is dependent upon the ability to visualise the tumour and as a result significant inter- and intra-clinician variability has been reported in the contouring of tumours of the prostate, lung, brain and oesophagus (Weltons et al., 2001; Steenbakkers et al., 2005).

The aim of the work presented in this case study was to develop a texture analysis methodology capable of distinguishing between the distinct pathology of the GTV and other clinically relevant regions on CT image data. For eight bladder patients (six male and two female), CT images were acquired at the radiotherapy planning stage and thereafter at regular intervals during treatment. All CT scans were acquired on a General Electric single slice CT scanner (IGE HiSpeed Fx/I, GE Medical Systems, Milwaukee, WI, USA). Seven patients were scanned with a 3 mm slice thickness and one patient with a 5 mm slice thickness. The repeat CT scans were registered against the corresponding planning reference CT scan to allow comparison of the same region on each image. Image features based on: the first-order histogram $(N = 7)$; second-order GTSDM $(N = 14)$; higher-order GLRLM $(N = 5)$; and a bespoke box-counting fractal approach $(N = 1)$ were calculated on pre-identified regions of the CT images of each patient (Nailon et al., 2008). Two classification environments were used to assess the performance of the approach in classifying the bladder, rectum and a region of multiple pathology on the axial, coronal and sagittal CT image planes. These were, in the first using all of the available features $(N = 27)$ and in the second using the best three features identified by the SFS approach. The classification results achieved are presented in Fig. 11. No significant discrimination was observed between the bladder, rectum and the region of multiple pathology on the axial, coronal and sagittal CT data using all of the available features $(N = 27)$. This is shown on the left column of Fig. 11. On the contrary, using the three best features identified by the SFS feature reduction approach, significant discrimination between the three pathological groups was possible. This is shown on the right column of Fig. 11. These results demonstrate the significant improvement in classification that can be achieved by removing features with little discriminatory power. Moreover the results demonstrate the effectiveness of texture analysis for classifying regions of interest, which may be difficult for the human observer to interpret.

The features that were found to work best were all from the GTSDM approach. The feature produced by the bespoke box-counting fractal approach was not found to have significant discriminatory power. However, more research is required into the use of fractal methods in this application area, particularly because assigning a single dimension to a whole region may not be appropriate (Mandelbrot, 1977). Furthermore, the fractal dimension calculation may have been influenced by the different distribution of grey-levels in the images due to variations in the amount of urine in the bladder and air in the rectum.

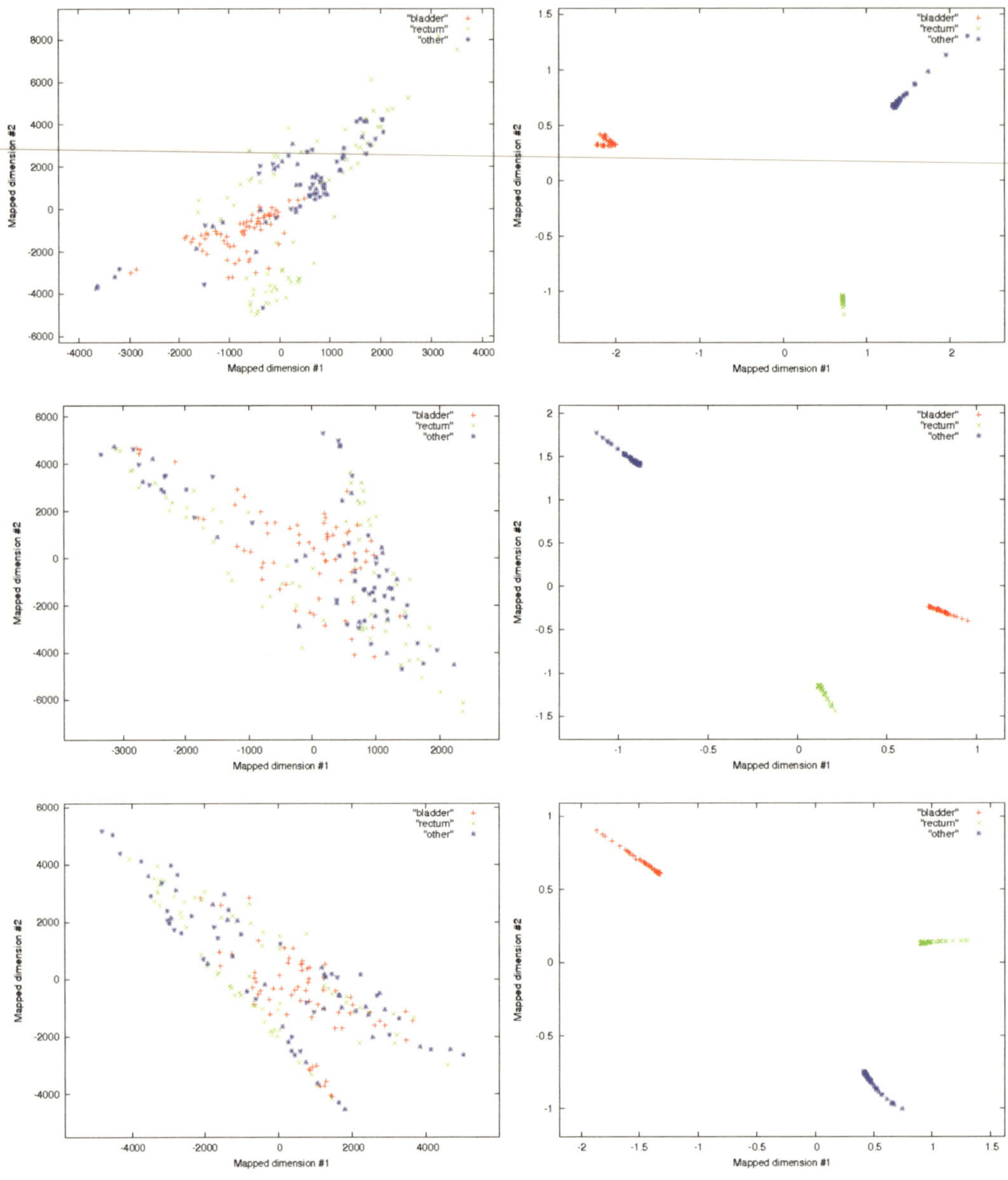

Fig. 11. Classification of the bladder, rectum and a region of multiple pathology identified as other on axial CT images through the pelvis using a texture analysis approach. Left (top: axial, middle: coronal, bottom: sagittal) plots showing the result of using all available features to classify the bladder, rectum and other. Right (top: axial, middle: coronal, bottom: sagittal) plots showing classification of the bladder, rectum and other using the best three features identified by the SFS approach. Sammon mapping was used to generate 2D representations of the multi-dimensional feature space and aid visualisation (Sammon, 1969).

The approach was also found to be insensitive to CT resolution and slice thickness for the data set studied. It was also noticed that discrimination of the bladder, rectum and other region in the coronal and sagittal image planes was comparable to the discrimination obtained in the axial plane. This is encouraging given that the coronal and sagittal data sets were produced from the axial data and suffer a loss of resolution because of finite CT slice thickness in the axial data acquisition procedure.

6.2 Case Study 2 – Prion Protein Characterisation Using Texture Analysis

Prion diseases are a group of fatal neurodegenerative diseases that occur in both animals and man (Bastian, 1991). Human prion diseases occur in sporadic, acquired and familial forms, the commonest of which is CJD (Ironside, 1998). The accumulation of prion protein within the brain is a cardinal feature of these diseases and can be identified by immunocytochemistry (Ironside et al., 2000). In this case study immunocytochemically stained sections were imaged using a Leica DMR microscope (Leica Microscopy Systems GmbH) and texture analysis techniques were applied to study the distribution of prion protein on the images acquired.

Formalin-fixed paraffin embedded tissue blocks were selected from the cerebellum of five cases of vCJD and seven cases of sporadic CJD with known codon 129 genotype and biochemical subtype (four cases of sporadic CJD methionine homozygotes type 1 and three cases of sporadic CJD methionine homozygotes type 2). From the blocks $5\mu m$ sections were cut and stained using the monoclonal antibody KG9 and lightly counterstained with haematoxylin. All images were acquired with 256 grey-levels using a $\times 10$ magnification factor on a 736×574 (pixel) frame (see Fig. 12). For each of the vCJD and sporadic CJD cases in the study cohort, 21 features (GTSDM = 9; GLRLM = 7; Fourier = 4; Fractal = 1) were calculated on eight neuropathologically significant regions of interest. Statistical analysis was performed on each feature using the Kruskal-Wallis test. This is a non-parametric test which makes no assumption about the distribution of the data (e.g. normality) and is used to compare three or more independent groups of sampled data. In this work the results were assessed at the 0.05 significance level. In addition, a Mann-Whitney test was used to assess the pair-wise discrimination between groups of sampled data. The hypothesis for the test was that the samples, or feature values, were significantly different between the groups being considered (Nailon et al., 2000).

The Kruskal-Wallis test showed that 18 of the 21 features were able to significantly differentiate between vCJD and sporadic CJD type 1 and 2 at the 0.05 significance level. The Mann-Whitney test, also at the 0.05 significance level, identified that 14 of the 21 features were able to significantly discriminate between the patterns of prion protein deposition found in vCJD and sporadic CJD type 1. The Mann-Whitney test also identified that 14 of the 21 features could significantly discriminate between vCJD and sporadic CJD type 2. It is interesting to note that the combination of GLRLM features found to be significant was different in the assessment of vCJD with sporadic CJD type 1 than vCJD with sporadic CJD type 2. This implies that different combinations of features may be required for different applications. The Mann-Whitney pair-wise significance test between sporadic CJD type 1 and type 2 found no features with significant discriminatory power. The results obtained in the study are summarised in Table 1.

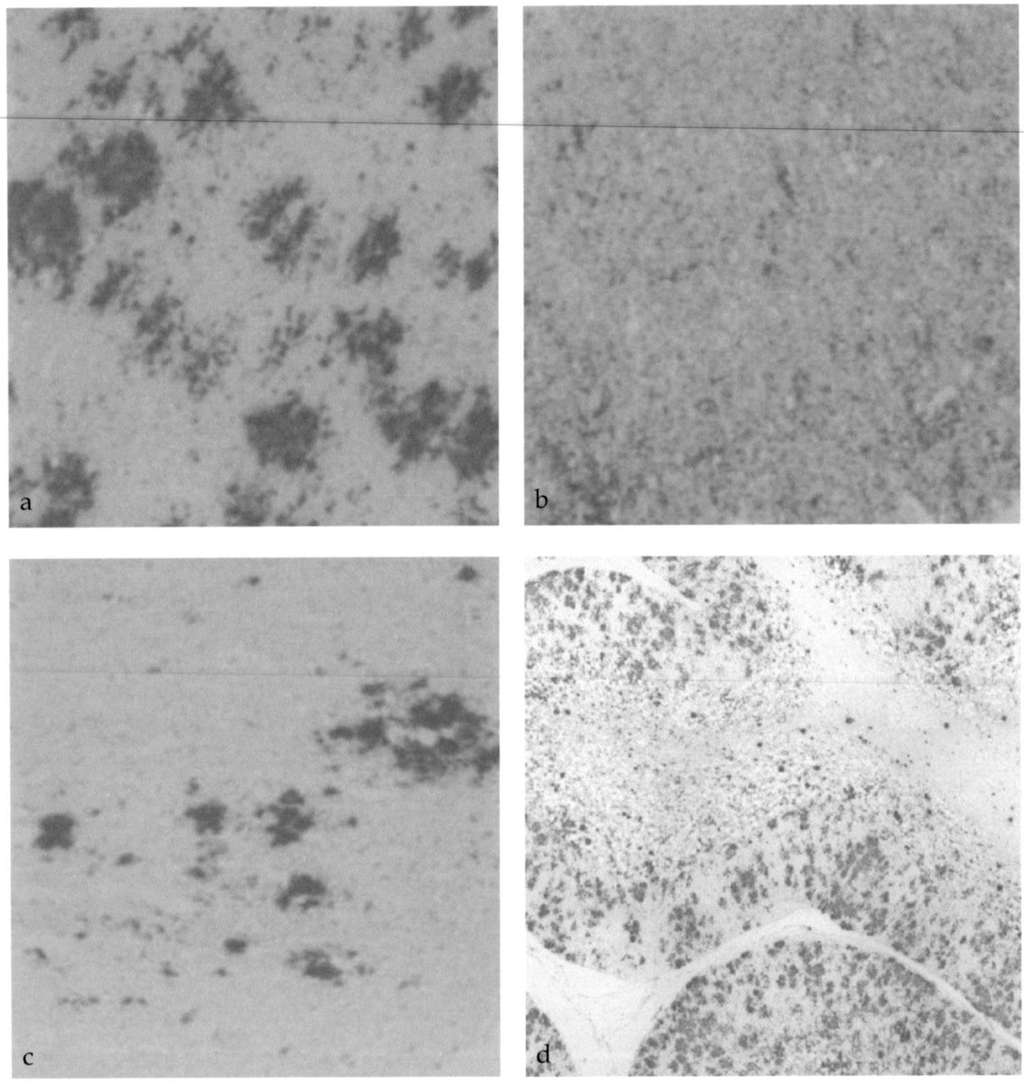

Fig. 12. Microscopic images showing the distribution of prion protein in the molecular layer of the cerebellum of cases of vCJD (a), sporadic CJD type 1 (b) and sporadic CJD type 2 (c). Figure d shows the distribution of prion protein in a larger region formed from nine overlapping microscopic images.

Feature	Method	Kruskall-Wallis		Mann-Whitney vCJD/spor CJD t1		Mann-Whitney vCJD/spor CJD t2		Mann-Whitney spor CJD t1/ spor CJD t2	
		Value	Power	Value	Power	Value	Power	Value	Power
f_1	GTSDM	0.052	-	0.556	-	0.071	-	0.057	-
f_2	GTSDM	0.005	+	0.111	-	0.036	+	0.057	-
f_3	GTSDM	0.004	+	0.016	+	0.036	+	1.000	-
f_4	GTSDM	0.050	+	0.111	-	0.143	-	0.114	-
f_5	GTSDM	0.000	+	0.016	+	0.036	+	0.057	-
f_6	GTSDM	0.004	+	0.016	+	0.036	+	0.857	-
f_7	GTSDM	0.002	+	0.016	+	0.036	+	0.400	-
f_8	GTSDM	0.007	+	0.016	+	0.571	-	0.571	-
f_9	GTSDM	0.061	-	0.016	+	0.786	-	0.400	-
f_{10}	GLRLM	0.020	+	0.111	-	0.143	-	0.057	-
f_{11}	GLRLM	0.065	-	0.111	-	0.250	-	0.114	-
f_{12}	GLRLM	0.000	+	0.016	+	0.036	+	0.057	-
f_{13}	GLRLM	0.050	+	0.111	-	0.143	-	0.114	-
f_{14}	GLRLM	0.050	+	0.111	-	0.143	-	0.114	-
f_{15}	GLRLM	0.000	+	0.016	+	0.036	+	0.114	-
f_{16}	GLRLM	0.001	+	0.032	+	0.036	+	0.057	-
f_{17}	Fourier (Ring 1)	0.002	+	0.016	+	0.036	+	0.400	-
f_{18}	Fourier (Ring 2)	0.002	+	0.016	+	0.036	+	0.400	-
f_{19}	Fourier (Ring 3)	0.002	+	0.016	+	0.036	+	0.400	-
f_{20}	Fourier (Ring 4)	0.002	+	0.016	+	0.036	+	0.400	-
f_{21}	Fractal	0.004	+	0.016	+	0.036	+	0.857	-

Table 1. Power of the features used to discriminate between: vCJD and sporadic CJD type 1; vCJD and sporadic CJD type 2; sporadic CJD type 1 and sporadic CJD type 2. The exact significance value is a measure of the discriminatory power of each feature. (+ indicates good discriminatory power, - indicates poor discriminatory power).

The choice of ring filters used was based on extensive trials on similar data sets. The radii of the final set of filters chosen is summarised in Table 2. The main objective of this work was to use texture analysis to investigate and study the distribution of prion protein found in vCJD and sporadic CJD. All of the Fourier ring features used showed significant discriminatory power in discriminating between vCJD and sporadic CJD types 1 and 2. However, they were unable to discriminate between sporadic CJD types 1 and 2.

Filter	Inner Radius	Outer Radius
1	$r_1 = 2$	$r_2 = 5$
2	$r_1 = 2$	$r_2 = 10$
3	$r_1 = 5$	$r_2 = 10$
4	$r_1 = 10$	$r_2 = 20$

Table 2. Inner and outer radii of the ring filters used to discriminate between: vCJD and sporadic CJD type 1; vCJD and sporadic CJD type 2; sporadic CJD type 1 and sporadic CJD type 2.

7. Summary

Texture analysis methods are useful for discriminating and studying both distinct and subtle textures in multi-modality medical images. Practical implementation requires careful consideration of the power of the individual features to discriminate between textures. This is essential to reduce the influence that heavily correlated features, and features with little discriminatory power, have on the overall classification. Statistical texture analysis techniques are constantly being refined by researchers and the range of applications is increasing. Fractal approaches, which offer the convenience of characterising a textured region by a single measure, appear more application-specific than statistical approaches and require more research. Algorithmic advances have been made on the use of full 3D texture analysis approaches and the publications in this area demonstrate that this is a promising area of research. This is particularly important given that biomedical image data with near isotropic resolution is becoming more common in clinical environments. However, it has been shown that there is minimal loss of discriminatory power when 2D techniques are applied in the coronal and sagittal planes.

8. Acknowledgements

The support of Dr. A.T. Redpath, Dr. D.B. McLaren and Professor S. McLaughlin is gratefully acknowledged for helpful discussion and preparation of the results presented in Case Study 1. I am also grateful to Professor J.W. Ironside and Dawn Everington for their assistance in obtaining the results presented in Case Study 2. The support of the laboratory staff at the National CJD Surveillance Unit, UK is acknowledged for preparation of the tissue samples used in Case Study 2. The support of the staff in the NHS Department of Oncology Physics and the School of Engineering at the University of Edinburgh is gratefully acknowledged. The James Clerk Maxwell Foundation is gratefully acknowledged for the provision of financial assistance to continue this work.

9. References

Bastian, F.O. (1991). Creutzfeldt-Jakob disease and other transmissible human spongiform encephalopathies. St Louis: Mosby Year Book.

Bajscy, R. (1973). Computer description of textured surfaces, *Proceedings of the Joint Conference on Artificial Intelligence*, August, pp. 572-579.

Brodatz, P. (1966). *Textures: a photographic album for artists and designers.* Dover Publications, ISBN 0-486-40699-7, New York.

Bruce, V.; Georgeson, M. & Green, P. (2003). *Visual Perception: Psychology and Ecology.* Psychology Press Publications, ISBN 1841692387, UK.

Conners, R. & Harlow, C. (1980). Theoretical comparison of texture algorithms. *IEEE Transactions on Pattern Analysis and Machine Intelligence*, Vol. 2, No. 3, pp. 204-222.

Devijver, P.A. & Kittler, J. (1982). *Pattern recognition: a statistical approach.* Prentice Hall, 0-13-654236-0, London.

Distani, R.; Nappi, M. & Riccio, D. (2006). A range/domain approximation error-based approach for fractal image compression. *IEEE Transactions on Image Processing*, Vol. 15, No. 1, pp. 89-97.

Duda, R.; Hart, P. & Stork, D. (2001). Pattern Classification, John Wiley & Sons, ISBN 0-471-05669-3.

Esgiar, A.; Naguib, R.; Sharif, B.; Bennet, M. & Murray, A. (2002). Fractal analysis in the detection of colonic cancer images. *IEEE Transactions on Information Technology in Biomedicine*, Vol. 6, No. 1, pp 54-58.

Feder, J. (1988). *Fractals.* Plenum Press, ISBN 0-306-42851-2, New York.

Galloway, M.M. (1975). Texture analysis using grey-level run lengths. *Computer Graphics and Image Processing*, Vol. 4, pp. 172-179.

Gonzalez, R.C. & Woods, R.E. (2001). *Digital Image Processing*, Prentice Hall, ISBN 0-201-18075-8.

Haralick, R.M.; Shanmugam K. & Dinstein, I. Texture features for image classification. *IEEE Transactions on Pattern Analysis and Machine Intelligence*, Vol. SMC-3, No. 6, Nov 1973, 610-621.

Hartigan, J. (1975). *Clustering Algorithms.* John Wiley & Sons, ISBN 0-471-35645-X.

ICRU, (1999). International Commission on Radiation Units and Measurements. ICRU Report 62: Prescribing, Recording and Reporting Photon Beam Therapy (Supplement to ICRU 50), Oxford University Press.

Ironside, J.W. (1998). Neuropathological findings in new variant Creutzfeldt-Jakob disease and experimental transmission of BSE. *FEMS Immunology & Medical Microbiology*, Vol. 21, No. 2, pp. 91-95.

Ironside, J.W.; Head, M.W.; Bell, J.E.; McCardle, L. & Will, R.G. (2000). Laboratory diagnosis of variant Creutzfeldt-Jakob disease, *Histopathology*, Vol. 37, No. 1, pp. 1-9.

Jain, A.K. & Chandrasekaran. (1982). Dimensionality and sample size considerations. In: *Pattern Recognition in Practice*, Krishnaiah, P.R. & Kanal, L.N., Vol. 2, pp. 835-888. North Holland.

Jain, A.K. & Zongker, D. (1997). Feature selection: evaluation, application and small sample performance. *IEEE Transactions on Pattern Analysis and Machine Intelligence*, Vol. 2, No. 19, pp. 153-158.

Julesz, B. (1975). Experiments in the visual perception of texture. *Scientific American*, Vol. 232, pp 34-43.

Kachouie, N. & Fieguth, P. (2007). A medical texture local binary pattern for TRUS prostate segmentation, *Proceedings of the 29th International Conference of the IEEE Engineering and Biology Society*, Lyon, France, August 23rd – 26th.

Karahaliou, A.; Boniatis, I; Skiadopoulos, S. & Sakellaropoulos, F. (2008). Breast cancer diagnosis: analyzing texture of tissue surrounding microcalcifications. *IEEE Transactions on Information Technology in Biomedicine*, Vol. 12, No. 6, pp. 731-738.

Kovalev, V.; Kruggel, F.; Gertz, H. & von Cramon D. (2001). Three-dimensional texture analysis of MRI brain datasets. *IEEE Transactions on Medical Imaging*, Vol. 20, No. 5, pp. 424-433.

Kurani, A.; Xu, D.; Furst, J. & Raicu, D. (2004). Co-occurrence matrices for volumetric data, *Proceedings of 7th IASTED International Conference on Computer Graphics and Imaging*, Kauai, Hawaii, USA, August 17th – 19th.

Li, L. & Qi, D. (2007) Detection of cracks in computer tomography images of logs based on fractal dimension, *Proceedings of the IEEE International Conference on Automation and Logistics*, pp. 2259-2264, Jinan China, August 18th - 21st .

Mandelbrot, B.B. (1977). *Fractals: form, chance and dimension.* W.H. Freeman and Co., ISBN 0-716-70473-0, New York.

Mirmehdi, M.; Xie, X. & Suri, J. (eds) (2008). *Handbook of texture analysis,* Imperial College Press, 1-84816-115-8, UK.

Meyer, J.L. (ed) (2007). *Frontiers of radiation therapy and oncology (vol 40): IMRT, IGRT, SBRT, advances in the treatment planning and delivery of radiotherapy*, Karger, 978-3-8055-9188 9, Switzerland.

Nailon, W.H. (1997). *Tissue characterisation of intravascular ultrasound using texture analysis.* Ph.D. dissertation, The University of Edinburgh, School of Engineering.

Nailon, W.H.; Everington, D. & Ironside, J.W. (2000). *Prion protein characterisation by image analysis.* Internal communication, National CJD Surveillance Unit, Edinburgh, UK.

Nailon, W.H. & Ironside, J.W. (2000) Variant Creutzfeldt-Jakob disease: immunocytochemical studies and image analysis. *Microscopy Research & Technique*, Vol. 50, No. 1, pp. 2-9.

Nailon, W.H.; Redpath, A.T. & McLaren, D.B. (2008). Characterisation of radiotherapy planning volumes using textural analysis. *Acta Oncologica*, Vol. 47, pp. 1303-1308.

Nouza, J. (1995). On the speech feature selection problem: are dynamic features more important than static ones? *Proceedings of the European Conference on Speech Communication and Technology*, pp 917-921, Madrid, Spain, September.

Peitgen, H. & Saupe, D. (1988). *The science of fractal images.* Springer-Verlag, ISBN 0-387-96608-0, New York.

Peitgen, H.; Jurgen, H. & Saupe, D. (1992). *Chaos and fractals: new frontiers of science.* Springer-Verlag, ISBN 0-387-97903-4, New York.

Pietikainen, M.K. (ed) (2000). *Texture analysis in machine vision*, World Scientific Publishing, 981-02-4373-1, Singapore.

Pentland, P. (1984). Fractal-based description of natural scenes. *IEEE Transactions on Pattern Analysis and Machine Intelligence*, Vol. PAMI-6, No. 6, Nov, pp. 661-674.

Podda, B.; Zanetti, G. & Giachetti, A. (2005). Texture analysis for vascular segmentation from CT images, *Proceedings of Computer Assisted Radiology and Surgery (CARS)*, pp. 206-211, Berlin, Germany, 22nd-25th June, 2005.

Pratt, W.K. (1978). *Digital Image Processing*, John Wiley & Sons, 0-471-01888-0, New York.

Press, W.; Flannery, B.; Teulkolsky, S. & Vetterling, W. *Numerical recipes in C: the art of scientific computing*. Cambridge University Press, ISBN 0-521-35465-X, UK.

Russ, J.C. (1994). *Fractal surfaces*. Plenum Press, ISBN 0-306-44702-9, New York.

Sammon, J. (1969). A nonlinear mapping for data structure analysis. *IEEE Transactions on Computing*, Vol, C-18, pp. 401-409.

Steenbakkers, R.J.H.M.; Duppen, J.C.; Fitton, I.; Deurloo, K.E.I.; Zijp, L.; Uitterhoeve A.L.J.; Rodrigus P.T.R.; Kramer, G.W.P.; Bussink, J.; De Jaeger, K.; Belderbos, J.S.A.; Hart, A.A.M.; Nowak, P.J.C.M.; van Herk, M. & Rasch, C.R.N. (2005). Observer variation in target volume delineation of lung cancer related to radiation oncologist-computer interaction: a 'big-brother' evaluation. *Radiotherapy & Oncology*, Vol. 77, pp. 182-190.

Stearns, S.D. (1976). On selecting features for pattern classifiers. *In Proceedings of the 3rd International Conference on Pattern Recognition*, pp. 71-75, Colorado, USA.

Stoyan, D. & Stoyan, H. (1994). *Fractals, random shapes and point fields: methods of geometrical statistics*. John Wiley & Sons, ISBN 0-471-93757-6, New York.

Therrien, C.W. (1989). *Decision estimation and classification: an introduction to statistical pattern recognition and related topics*, John Wiley & Sons, 0-471-83102-6, New York.

Tuceryan, M. & Jain, A.K. (1998). Texture analysis. In: Chen, C.H; Pau, L.F. & Wang, P.S.P., (eds). *The handbook of pattern recognition and computer vision*. 2nd ed. World Scientific Publishing Co., ISBN 9-810-23071-0, Singapore.

Turcotte, D.L. (1992). *Fractals and Chaos in Geology and Geophysics*, Cambridge University Press, ISBN 0-521-56164-7, Cambridge, UK.

Uppaluri, R.; Mitsa, T.; Sonka, M.; Hoffman, E. & McLennan G. (1997). Quantification of pulmonary emphysema from lung computed tomography images. *American Journal of Respiratory Care in Medicine*, Vol. 156, No. 1, pp. 248-254.

Weber, A.G. (2004). The USC texture mosaics. *University of Southern California Viterbi School of Engineering*, http://sipi.usc.edu/ .

Weltons, C.; Menten, J.; Feron, M.; Bellon, E.; Demaerel, P.; Maes, F.; van den Bogaert, W. & van der Schueren, E. (2001). Interobserver variations in gross tumor volume delineation of brain tumours on CT and impact of MRI. Radiotherapy & Oncology, Vol. 60, No. 1, pp. 49-59.

Winzenrieth, R. & Claude, I. (2006). Is there functional vascular information in anatomical MR sequences? A preliminary in vivo study. *IEEE Transactions on Biomedical Engineering*, Vol. 53, No. 6, June 2006, pp.1190-1194.

Xu, D.; Kurani, A. & Raicu, D. (2004). Run-length encoding for volumetric texture, *Proceedings of 4th IASTED International Conference on Visualization, Imaging and Image Processing – VIIP*, Marbella, Spain, September 6th – 8th.

Xu, Y.; Sonka, G.; McLennan, G.; Junfeng, G. & Hoffman, E. (2006). MDCT-based 3D texture classification of emphysema and early smoking related pathologies. *IEEE Transactions on Medical Imaging*, Vol. 25, No. 4, pp. 464-475.

Yu, H.; Caldwell, C.; Mah, K. & Mozeg D. (2009). Co-registered FDG PET/CT based textural characterization of head and neck cancer in radiation treatment planning. *IEEE Transactions on Medical Imaging*, Vol. 28, No. 3, pp. 374-383.

Yu, Z.; Jixian, Z. & Haitao, L. (2007). Fractal characteristics of very high resolution satellite imagery, *Proceedings of Geoscience and Remote Sensing Symposium*, pp. 389-92, Barcelona, Spain, July 23rd-27th.

Zhou, B.; Xuan, J.; Zhao, H.; Chepko, M.; Freedman, M. & Yingyin, K. (2007). Polarization imaging for breast cancer diagnosis using texture analysis and svm, Proceedings of Life Sciences Systems and Applications Workshop, pp. 217-220, Bethesda, Maryland, USA.

Zonger, D. & Jain, A. (1996). Algorithms for feature selection: an evaluation. *Proceedings of the 13th International Conference on Pattern Recognition (ICPR'96)*, Vol. B, pp. 18-22, Vienna, Austria, August.